A Magical Guide to

Love & Sex

A Magical Guide to
Love & Sex

CASSANDRA EASON

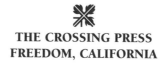

THE CROSSING PRESS
FREEDOM, CALIFORNIA

For information on bulk purchases or group discounts for this and other Crossing Press titles, please contact our Special Sales Director at 800/777-1048, ext. 203.

Visit our Web site: **www.crossingpress.com**

Library of Congress Cataloging-in-Publication Data

Eason, Cassandra.
    A magical guide to love & sex : how to use rituals, spells, and nature's energies to bring love into your life / Cassandra Eason.
        p. cm.
    Originally published: London : J. Piatkus, 2000.
    Includes bibliographical references and index.
    ISBN 1-58091-107-2 (pbk.)
    1. Magic. 2. Love--Miscellanea. 3. Sex--Miscellanea.   I. Title:
Magical guide to love and sex. II. Title: Love & sex. III. Title.
    BF1623.S4 E27 2001
    133.4'42--dc21
                                    2001047255

0   9   8   7   6   5   4   3   2   1

Contents

Introduction: When Will I Find Love?   1

1 The History of Love and Fertility   15

2 Attracting Love   25

3 The Plants of Love   43

4 Dreaming of Love   62

5 Fidelity and Lasting Love   86

6 The Fertility of the Earth   109

7 Love Divination   126

8 Ending Love   143

9 The Festivals of Love and Fertility   160

10 Twin Souls   189

11 Sex Magic   206

Appendix: A Treasury of Love   225

When Will I Find Love?

My true love has my heart and I have his,
By just exchange, one for the other given,
I hold his dear and mine he cannot miss,
There never was a better bargain driven,
He loves my heart for once it was his own,
I cherish his, because in me it bides—

from 'The Bargain' by Sir Philip Sidney

The idealistic images of Elizabethan poet Sir Philip Sidney have inspired would-be lovers over the centuries; even in our own less poetic times, many of us yearn for a soul mate who will enhance our life on a spiritual as well as mental and physical level, share our joys and encourage and support us through difficulties. This book is for those in love and those who seek love, for those wishing to strengthen and deepen existing relationships and for those hoping to attract a new lover, whether for the first time or after sorrow and the failure of an earlier relationship.

There is someone for each one of us, perhaps not the handsome prince or fairy tale princess, the sex god in the gym or the heiress with the unquenchable libido, but a kindred spirit who will make us happy, will be loyal and loving through the mundane and sorrowful times, as well as the fields of flowers and perpetual sunshine. It may be someone you know already, a dear friend, or a person who will suddenly enter your life from across the world and change your universe in an instant. Love is unpredictable and may strike at the least likely time and in the most unromantic place.

Over the course of the book I explore in detail many aspects of love and relationships, the concept of twin souls, of sacred sexuality, sex magic, dreaming of love, divination for love and the secret language of lovers; above all I focus on love at its most natural and spontaneous, the innate ability we have to attract the right mate, to remain together for many years and perhaps to have children. Love and virility do not need complex manuals, but follow the natural energies of the year: the spring of awakening feelings towards your chosen partner, the summer of consummation and commitment, and the autumn and winter of fulfilment and mature love, or love second or even third time around, wiser and more fruitful in that knowledge.

Love rituals are as old as time itself, with feelings and desires focused through herbs, flowers, the sunshine, moonlight and fertilising rain. But like our forebears, it is important to know what it is we are asking of the cosmos and Mother Earth in our spell-casting. Love magic is very potent and cannot be used to bind people against their will or make a person love you and leave someone else, without consequences that need careful consideration, on both an earthly and magical level. Love magic should always be performed without malice, however justifiable the negative feelings, for hope attracts hope; love even in loss will radiate outwards and like all magic return its blessings – and malevolence – threefold.

Love magic can add passion to an existing relationship and encourage fidelity; what is more, the old ways can sometimes boost fertility, by reconnecting with the ancient earth energies and festivals of the natural world that linked our ancestors' fertility with that of the land itself. Equally, if you are with someone who makes you unhappy, love magic can give you the strength to walk away from a destructive relationship, or if there is the possibility of a reconciliation, to banish anger and resentment so that a new, stronger bond can grow.

We all need to be loved, but may lack confidence in our own worth or have suffered loss and betrayal. It can be hard, if you are lonely or feel your biological clock is ticking, to wait for that special person without seeking love to the exclusion of all other thoughts or, if found, worrying about how long it will last. This doubt is natural, especially if you have been hurt in love or feel that the right partner eludes you. Even the most beautiful or handsome movie stars, foot-ballers or pop singers can have a series of disastrous love affairs if the inner person sees themself as ugly and unworthy of love.

Love begins with the self. If you do not love yourself, you have no touchstone against which to measure the love of others, and may unconsciously seek a 'perfect' partner to compensate for your own perceived inadequacies and fears – and then be disillusioned when the idol has feet of clay. Worse still, you may accept less than loving treatment because you feel you are not worth more. It has taken me almost fifty years and several failed relationships to begin to accept that love is a precious gift rather than a favour or obligation that demands selfless sainthood or living by another's rules. Instead of asking *What is wrong with me?*, ask *How can I best open myself to loving energies in every aspect of my life, so that when the right person comes along I shall be ready to share myself and accept the other person as he or she truly is?*

The following love ritual involves yourself alone, whether you are in a close relationship, have many lovers or are single by choice or necessity, and is a reminder of how special you are.

(

Enhancing Self-Love and Self-Esteem

+ First, make a bath of love, as if you are preparing for a very special date. If possible, carry out the ritual on a Friday, the day of Venus, Goddess of love, and at her hour, the third hour after sunset; or at dawn on a Friday when the sunlight is first breaking through.

+ The basic ingredients for your love infusion are (per bath tub of water) one and a half tablespoons of Epsom salts (magnesium sulphate), one tablespoon of baking powder (bicarbonate of soda) and half a tablespoon of sea salt. Alternatively, use commercially made bath salts with essential oils already added.

+ If you have bought bath salts, mix them as though you are creating them. Blend the ingredients together in a glass or ceramic bowl with a wooden or ceramic spoon, saying as a mantra:

I am beautiful in my own eyes, I am worthy of love, I am complete in myself.

+ Add an essential oil of love to the salts; between six and ten drops of one of the following mild oils is ideal: geranium, lavender, rose or ylang-ylang. With each drop, say: *I am as I am and that is good.*

✦ Light six pink candles (the number and colour of Venus) in a safe place in the bathroom, saying:

Light one for acceptance of those parts of myself that I cannot change,

Light two for healing past wounding words that diminish my self-esteem,

Light three to enhance what I, not others, seek to change about myself,

Light four for the knowledge that I am essentially lovable and attractive to those known and unknown to me who may bring me happiness,

Light five for the potential love and joy waiting along my life path if I allow it to unfold in its own time,

Light six for the ability to give freely of my approval and admiration of others, knowing that what is given without condition returns threefold.

✦ Make sure the candles cast pools of light into the water as you start to run your bath, saying to the rhythm of the flow of the water:

Love flow to me, flow this night,
Venus, Star of love shine bright.

Or at dawn, say:

Love flow to me, flow this morn,
Venus, Star of love and dawn.

✦ When the bath is full, turn off the taps and light six sticks or cones of jasmine or neroli incense around the bathroom, naming one of your virtues or strengths with each, for example:

I light this incense for my ability not to make a drama out of a crisis/to find solutions when everyone else despairs.

✦ Next, scatter in your love salt a handful at a time, if possible into a pool of candlelight. With each handful, circle the water nine times, saying:

Love ripples spread and circle, as I give freely my love to myself and in doing so to others, knowing even if this love is not returned immediately, that my power thereby is increased, three times three.

✦ Lie in the bath, gazing at the ripples of light in the water, and see the radiance entering every pore of your body.

✦ When you are ready, dry yourself and wash the water down the plug hole with a few drops of cleansing pine oil, saying:

Doubts and fears, flow to the sea
Never more to trouble me
Many loves will come my way
Those I love, will choose to stay.

As with so many rituals, this has incorporated the four ancient elements of Earth (the salt), Air (the incense), Fire (the candle) and Water (the oil and bath water). It was believed that if you united these four elements, a fifth, ether or akasha, greater than the others would result from the union and magical energies thereby be released.

Creating Love Rituals

The four elements were represented by flowers, herbs, fires and flowing water in the natural magic practised by our ancestors to bring love and fertility into their lives. These old rituals and the seasonal events that formed a natural focus are discussed in greater detail in 'The Festivals of Love and Fertility'. It is only as we have moved away from the natural cycles of life to a world of artificial lighting and heating, cultivation and transportation systems that magic has needed books or teachers apart from grandmothers or the village wise ones. But even today, the best love and fertility spells are those devised by yourself at a time of need, using the words that come from your heart, for emotions and desires are a strong impetus for magic.

Throughout this book the words and mantras used are either traditional or those that I or other practitioners have found helpful. You may wish to begin to loose-leaf folder or special notebook in which you write down your favourite spells and any materials, herbs or crystals that you discover. In the back of this book I have given some common associations for candle colours, crystals, herbs, and so on, but if these do not work for you, try others. There are so many magical traditions for it is at essence an interactive art that grows and evolves, and I also use one or two 'techno-spells' as well as the ancient love charms so beloved of our ancestors. A spell can be simple or complex, according to the desired outcome, but you need to specify its parameters. You also need a specific focus, whether candles in appropriate zodiacal colours for yourself and a lover (see page 238), a tiny doll for a much desired baby, a silver heart for new love or a ring for marriage, silver being the colour and metal of the Moon, which is in itself linked to love and fertility.

Recently, I have come to appreciate the significance of giving a spell a time limit in some instances, though in other cases you need to be more flexible. If, for example, you ask to be married within three months or become pregnant within two months, you may be precluding exciting plans in store for you at a later date or the fact that it might not be the right time to have a baby. However, if you wanted to begin a spell on the New Moon and use increasing or waxing energies, perhaps to give a quick boost to a faltering love affair, you might concentrate the power by saying:

This spell shall cease to hold its sway
When the Full Moon has passed its day.

You can also focus the new energies over, say, a period of three days, by using a candle with three wicks and repeating the ritual centred around a new flame each day.

Creating a Love or Fertility Amulet

Whether you seek love or fertility, you can create a powerful token or amulet and charge it with your personal energies and emotions, thereby giving it extra potency. Jewellery is a good focus for such powers as it is bright and thereby naturally attracts positive forces. And because it is worn on your body, you are constantly in touch with its energies.

For love, a silver locket or a clear crystal earring set in silver is ideal; real crystal is best. For fertility, the adornment should be something oval, perhaps an amber pendant, an organic gem said to contain the power of many suns set in its own metal, gold for the Sun or a moonstone in silver. An emerald ring, bracelet or pendant with even a tiny stone is Venus's special jewel, symbol of fidelity and fertility; worn on the heart finger or close to the heart, it will have special potency.

Rings and bracelets in general signify love without end and a willingness to remain true to another. Plain gold or silver will serve if it is not appropriate to wear gems – and a gift from a lover is best of all.

CHARGING YOUR PERSONAL LOVE
OR FERTILITY AMULET

At the Full Moon, take your love or fertility symbol into the moonlight. If it is a cloudy night you can carry out the ritual up to two nights later, or light a huge silver candle outdoors and focus on that instead.

From Neolithic times the three phases of the Moon – waxing, full and waning – were regarded as representing the maiden, mother and wise woman or crone stages of woman-hood respectively. So the Full Moon is associated with the full power of love, the consummation of that love, and with fertility, for it was believed that the Moon Mother took souls into her womb after death and allowed them to be reborn. So the Full Moon offers great potency for any love or fertility amulet which, once charged with power, becomes a talisman able to attract what is sought. You can use this method with other love and fertility charms.

✦ Fill a silver-coloured dish with water and add a sprinkling of sea salt.

✦ Position the bowl so that the moonlight or candlelight is within the water, and with your amulet in your power hand (the one you write with), use your other hand to splash six drops of water on the jewellery saying:

Earth and Water, charge this symbol of my love/fertility with the gentle nourishment and growth of Mother Earth, with the flow of the rivers that becomes the ebb and flow of the tides, to be drawn upwards and to fall as gentle rain once more, nourishing the soil in the never ceasing cycle of growth and new life from old.

✦ Hold your amulet so that it sparkles in the moonlight and turn it over six times, saying six times for love:

Moon of love, Moon of delight,
As this jewel fills with light
May I draw such love to me,
That I with joy may radiant be.

For fertility, say six times:

Mother Moon, maternal might,
Fill now my womb with fertile light
As you are full, so may I be
New life to grow and wax in me.

Wear your charged symbol and it will make you more charismatic in every way; whether you are seeking commitment or to conceive a child, the powers of nature within the charm will amplify your innate powers of attraction and fertility.

You can rededicate your symbol on each Full Moon, and each day you wear it and make wishes for your future, it will absorb your desires and grow in power.

How Do Love and Fertility Spells Work?

There are two basic kinds of spell: attracting and banishing. Attracting spells work on the principle of either sympathetic or contagious magic, which are remarkably similar. Sympathetic magic works on the principle that the symbol of, for example, a lover or baby is affected magically by building up energies through chants or rhymes repeated with increasing speed and intensity. When these energies are concentrated, they can be released in a final chant or action into the cosmos, so drawing power from the unseen to the seen world. You might release a kite or balloon to whose string you have attached your wishes, tie coloured scarves in knots and then release the energy either immediately or when you need the power, dance faster and faster as you chant until you finally fling your arms in the air with a cry. You would do to the symbol what you wish to happen to the person it represents, for example, incubating a doll in an egg shell from the New to the Full Moon, and when the Moon was Full, pricking the egg with a needle to symbolise the coming together of male/female energies, and on the same night making love in the moonlight on the principle that like attracts like.

Contagious magic is even more direct and uses something connected with the person you wish to attract, for example, a lock of hair, an article of clothing, perfume or aftershave, or even the soil in which he or she has made a footprint. Many early countryside spells followed this principle, with a couple making love in the fields to make the corn grow and at the same time, by direct contact, transferring the fertility of the soil to themselves.

When you wish to end a relationship or to lessen the power of a destructive relationship, you should never attempt to banish a person, only his or her negative hold. You might bind together two dolls and then cut the knot, light two candles from a single flame to mark the separation of two people, write your regrets on paper and burn them in a candle flame, cast a symbolic stone or flower into a fast-flowing stream, releasing the negativity, or bury a token of the broken love. You can dispose of any leftover candle wax and other material from your rituals either by burying them in a biodegradable container if the items will decompose naturally, or simply in a paper bag with your rubbish, remembering to add a pinch of salt for cleansing. Some people keep the workings until the spell of either attraction or banishing is fulfilled in the external world, but I find it is better to mark an ending and if necessary begin with new ingredients and fresh hope.

Psychic Protection

If you work with only good intent and never try to curse or harm another person by thought or deed, however much they may have maligned or betrayed you, you carry inbuilt protection. Nevertheless, it can be good to mark the beginning of a ritual and to close down psychic energies afterwards. There are many methods you can use and I have given a number of these in my book *The Complete Guide to Magic and Ritual* (Piatkus, 1999).

☽

CREATING SENTINELS OF LIGHT

The following method is my favourite. Circles create a sacred space that offers power and protection. You can draw a physical one on the ground in chalk or crayon or visualise a circle of light by drawing one in the air waist-high with a crystal. In either case, begin in the north in one single unbroken movement in a clockwise direction, whether the circle is actual or visualised.

Round the edge of your actual or visualised circle, set candles at the four main compass positions. Some people see these candles as angels or Archangels. At the end of a spell, thank your guardians and uncast the circle in the opposite direction, anti-clockwise, either rubbing it out if you actually drew a circle, or gradually seeing the light fade from a visualised one. You can blow out the protective candles first, but I prefer to leave them burning until last and then send the light into the universe or towards those who have hurt you.

You need only light your protective candles periodically. On other occasions you can invoke the candle protection without lighting them. If you are in a hurry or it is not possible to use candles, use the following simple ritual:

✦ Position a tall white candle in each of the four main compass positions around the room or around a table where you are working, so that you are sitting or standing inside their protective circle whether or not you created a magic circle. Make sure you can move safely without burning yourself on the candles. In the summer you could use outdoor candles, perhaps in a protective fragrance such as citronella (which is also excellent for repelling insects), and make a really big working area, perhaps with a tree stump to hold your magical objects.

✦ As dusk falls, light the Candle of the North. As you light it say:

Candle of the North, encircle me with the power of the Earth, the strength of ancient stone circles, tall craggy mountains and high stone walls that I may work safe within your light.

✦ Visualise light radiating from the flame and forming a brilliant laser beam eastwards in an arc extending to the Candle of the East.

✦ Light the Candle of the East, saying:

Candle of the East, encircle me with the power of mighty winds that I may be safe within the eye of the storm.

✦ Visualise its beam forming an arc of light extending southwards until it touches the Candle of the South.

◆ Light the Candle of the South, saying:

Candle of the South, surround me with protective fire that once stood sentinel on hilltops driving away darkness and negative power that would do harm.

◆ Visualise its light rays extending to the Candle of the West.

◆ Finally, light the Candle of the West, saying:

Candle of the West, make me an island sanctuary that I may work in peace, surrounded by your protective waters, too deep and wide for any to cross with malice.

◆ Visualise its light moving northwards to form an unbroken circle of light.

◆ Make a gesture as you stand bathed in light, for example drawing a circle on your palm and saying:

When I make this sign when I am carrying out a ritual, my inner candles will instantly erect my protective barrier of light around me and those who share my spell.

◆ Blow out the candles, beginning in the West and proceeding anti-clockwise. Watch the circle of light fade, but not disappear. The candle guardians can be activated whenever you need them, but you should renew the protective circle regularly by lighting the candles and re-creating the circle.

◆ Once a month, on or close to the night of the Full Moon, light the four candles and leave them to burn right out in a safe place.

The History of Love and Fertility

L ove magic began in the form of fertility rites for the survival of the race. This is not to say that our ancestors did not feel or experience devotion, affection or desire; we may surmise that they gave flowers, exchanged tokens of love and perhaps even made vows under the stars. But what have survived as evidence from early pre-literate societies are ancient stone figurines that celebrated and also stimulated fertility in a woman and the animals on whom tribes depended for food, by a process of sympathetic magic. This chapter examines strands of history and folk lore that forms the roots of modern love and fertility magic, and which may still offer answers to dilemmas that the modern world cannot resolve or, in some cases, has created as close contact with the soil has diminished. For though the mechanics of sex and the physical aspects of attraction appear in every newspaper and magazine, and advances in the medical field of physiological infertility have been immense, what has been lost is the connection with the natural cycles of the seasons and the joy and spontaneity of lovemaking.

In the early hunter-gatherer societies the Earth Mother was worshipped as the giver of all life and fertility, and so menstruation, pregnancy and childbirth were likewise regarded as sacred. The Venus of Willendorf, the earliest fertility figurine, dates from around 24,000–22,000 BC and is made of limestone. She is just over 11cm (4.5 in) high, with voluptuous breasts, buttocks and thighs, a deliberately emphasised genital area and a swollen stomach. As with similar figures she has no face and rows of plaited hair are wrapped around her head. A particular characteristic of Palaeolithic Venus figurines is the lack of feet. It may have been that such images were intended to be held in the hand as a fertility token, and some have seen her role as a talisman in childbirth, perhaps alleviating pain as women called out to the Mother in their labour.

Twenty-five thousand years ago, Palaeolithic people saw man and nature as inextricably linked and acknowledged the life force as deities in every rock, tree, stream and primarily in the Earth herself. Having been formerly discredited as simplistic, this animistic view is now increasingly recognised as being true on the deepest spiritual level. Sympathetic magic was used to invoke these deities and mating rituals were enacted to persuade the herds to produce offspring and also milk. The fertility statuettes may have served as a focus for these fertility rites, carried from place to place as the tribes followed the herds.

Because the hunt was of prime importance and the food source usually consisted of horned and fierce animals, the early God of hunting was depicted as horned. By Neolithic times the hunter-gatherer culture gave way to agriculture and the God evolved into the son/consort of the Earth Mother, God of vegetation/corn/winter and death, who offered himself in sacrifice each year and was reborn at the Mid-winter Solstice as the son/Sun God. The horn and its obvious association with the phallus became a symbol of male potency and courage, but still recognised the sanctity of the woman as the giver of life. This male potency symbol has survived the passage of time in such festivals as the annual Abbots Bromley Horn Dance in September and in ancient bull worship traditions. As the sky gods gained supremacy over the Earth Mother, tall pillar stones and towers as well as small phallic stones made of jade or precious metals were created and many of these monuments and towers were linked with the sexual potency of the sun and sky gods; the biblical tower of Babel, for example, may have been the great Ziggurat in Babylon, described by the Greek Herodotus in 450 BC as having a temple to Marduk the Babylonian Supreme God at the top, in which noblewomen lay on a golden couch to have intercourse with the God on His descent from heaven. But with the coming of Christianity, the Horned God became demonised as Satan and open phallic worship was regarded as evil. Phallic stones, such as the one at Cerne Abbas, were destroyed by missionaries like St Augustine, though amazingly the chalk Giant survived.

The Neolithic period also saw the development of shrines to the Triple Goddess who became associated with the three phases of the Moon – waxing, full, and waning. These lunar stages echoed the monthly female cycle with peak fertility at the Full Moon. Indeed, women may have routinely bled at the dark of the Moon and so mirrored Moon cycles exactly. Hence the Full Moon was associated with romance and passion, and Moon magic for the increase of love and fertility is still practised under the auspices of the waxing Moon.

As civilisations evolved so the importance of fertility became linked to the continuation of the blood line, an increasingly significant factor as both titles and property required an unbroken link of descent to prevent wars when one leader died; this affected even those who had the humblest dwelling or tools to pass on to a new generation.

In Ancient Egypt, because the Nile was so important for the fertility of the land when it flooded, Nile creatures such as the fish, the hippopotamus and the crocodile were also regarded as deities of human fertility. Heket, a frog, was revered as the Goddess of childbirth, as was Tauret, Taueret or Tawaret, the hippopotamus Goddess, who ruled over conception, pregnancy and safe childbirth. The importance of female fertility to the Ancient Egyptians is also demonstrated by the numerous clay, wooden or stone images of nude women that have been excavated, with the pubic triangle clearly marked. Such figurines were also offered to Hathor, Goddess of wisdom and music, who was closely connected with sexuality, fertility and childbirth, probably with requests for children or as thanks for a safe birth. The Egyptian Isis/Horus statues also celebrated woman as the mother, and are linked with the later European Black Madonna statues, themselves powerful fertility icons. After reassembling the body of her husband Osiris after his murder and dismemberment, Isis impregnated herself on his magical phallus, so ensuring the continuation of the blood line of the gods with the birth of Horus.

The Celts had their own fertility figurines that survived into the Middle Ages and are still sometimes used by modern Wiccan women in childbirth. Sheelagh-na-gig is an abstract Celtic figure of a hag-like female form, probably the crone form of Brigit or Brigid the Triple Goddess. She indicates her enlarged genitals with her hands and holds her vulva open as though she is about to give birth. This is not as strange as it sounds, given the belief of the evolving trinity of goddesses. In the Celtic tradition the king or chieftain would ritually mate with the old hag of winter, who on his first embrace would turn into the maiden goddess once more. With Christianisation, Brigid became the late fifth-century St Bride or Brigit of Kildare and was in legend, though not in chronology, said to be the midwife of Christ. And as Mary replaced the mother goddesses, so were wayside shrines to St

Bride and to Mary herself adorned with fertility offerings – and sometimes with tiny booties when prayers had been answered.

The Virgin Mary, especially in the Middle Ages, retained a quasi-magical role in relation to marriage and childbirth. In *Un Normand*, a story by Guy du Maupassant, he tells of a shrine near Rouen known as Notre Dame du Gros Ventre (Our Lady of the Big Belly), which was highly regarded by young unmarried mothers-to-be. It was in the care of an eccentric character who composed his own prayer for the pregnant pilgrims. It began: 'Our good lady, the Virgin Mary, natural patron of girl-mothers in this country, protect your servant who slipped up in a moment of forgetfulness.' The prayer, which was strictly forbidden by the Church, ended: 'Do not forget me, above all alongside your holy husband and intercede with God the father that he might find me a husband as good as yours.'

Fertility rituals, albeit overlaid with love and courting aspects, continued in the countryside into the twentieth century. Young people would go out into the fields on May Eve and make love, while corn dollies and straw effigies woven from the previous year's corn were burned ritually and scattered on the fields to bring fertility to land and people alike (see 'The Festivals of Love and Fertility').

For though there were centuries of love poems dedicated to a maiden's rosy cheeks, her dulcet tones and honeyed eyes and the 'marriage of true minds' as Shakespeare expressed it, until the advent of sanitation and a sharp drop in infant mortality after the First World War the need to have many children was still vital in caring for elderly relatives. The Welfare State and the National Health Service were post-Second World War creations – and with them, for the working classes at least, came the finer points of courtship.

In Alhama de Almeria in Andalucia the old traditions

linger even today. Here, the Feast of the baby Jesus (El Nino Jesus) is held on Easter Sunday. The best bunch of grapes of the harvest is hung around the neck of the image of baby Jesus, which is carried around the village while the public struggle to get hold of the grapes; this is a direct descendant from the ancient fertility ceremonies.

But continuing the blood line was far from a young girl's thoughts as she dreamed of getting married and looked into the future to divine when she should be wed. Christian saints' days became the focus of these divinatory prayers and rites for young unmarried maidens and took on magical rather than religious significance. For example, on St Agnes Eve, January 20, or the following night of the actual Saint's day, young women have, since medieval times, practised love divination. Agnes is the patron saint of virgins and betrothed couples and suffered martyrdom under the Emperor Diocletian in the year AD 306 because she had dedicated herself to chastity and refused to compromise her faith.

On St Agnes Eve young girls, having fasted all day, should take a row of pins stuck into a square of paper or cloth and pull them out one after the other, saying a *pater noster* (The Lord's Prayer) for each, then fasten one pin at a time to the sleeve of their nightgowns. As they get into bed they recite:

Sweet Agnes work thy fast,
If ever I be to marry man
Or ever man to marry me
I hope this night him to see

Thus they are promised a dream of the man they will marry.

In the northern counties of England and Scotland the girl recites a rhyme rather than a *pater noster* with each pin, and asks the good saint that she will see her love in actuality the next day:

Fair St Agnes play the part,
And send to me my own sweetheart
Not in his best nor worst array
But in the clothes he wears each day
That tomorrow I may him ken
From among all other men.

St Catherine, the fourth-century patron saint of young women, whose name graces the main boulevard in Montreal, also inspired maidenly prayers for many centuries. On her feast day, November 25, young spinsters would go and pray for a husband in St Catherine's Chapel in the Abbey at Abbotsbury, Dorset:

A husband, St Catherine
A handsome one, St Catherine.
A rich one, St Catherine.
A nice one, St Catherine,
And soon, St Catherine.

Such a ritual was common wherever her chapel existed. For example, in the grounds of the churchyard next to the sacred well at the ruined Abbey at Cerne Abbas in Dorset is a sacred well above which the Chapel of St Catherine formerly stood. At this spot, which is also a fertility well, and at the foot of the path to the phallic Cerne Abbas Giant, young girls would turn round three times clockwise and ask St Catherine for a husband, making the sign of the cross on their foreheads with the water which even today is safe to drink in spring when the flow is fast. Those who had their wishes instantly granted would then go up to the Giant to make love.

On St Mark's Eve, April 24, midnight was the hour for magic – the witching hour – and if a maiden set a supper table at midnight in silence, the wraith of her husband or his spirit double would sit down to dine and she might identify him. Peering through each church window in turn at midnight also promised a vision of the lover's face through the last window.

Pluck red sage leaves one at each stroke of midnight and the lover will appear.

Scatter ash on the hearth on the first stroke of midnight and the lover's footprint will be there in the morning.

Finally, and less aesthetically pleasing, the watching of the farthing candle also took place on St Mark's Eve. A group of young men or women would place a lighted stolen pig's tail on the floor. When the tail turned blue, each present would see their future husband or wife.

Scotland has its time of love on St Andrew's Eve, November 29, or the actual night of the 30th when at the stroke of midnight a maid should take hold of the latch of the door and call out three times: 'Gentle love if thou lovest me show thyself.' She then opens the door a few inches, snatches out into the dark and will find in her hand a lock of hair. It will belong to her true love. She must be alone in the house and tell no one what she does.

Alternatively, two girls sit in a room at midnight without speaking and each must take as many hairs from her head as she is years old. Having put them in a linen cloth with a herb called True love or Trillium (which, in infusion, when rubbed on to the body will attract love), as soon as the clock strikes one, they turn every hair separately, saying:

I offer this my sacrifice
To him most precious in my eyes,
I charge thee now come forth to me
That I this minute may thee see.

In the days before dating agencies and equality, when women could not proposition a man openly, these charms opened the way for lovers to be drawn together by fate. If taken seriously, they offered choices of lovers who might have been rejected or not considered on a conscious level, but in astral form suddenly became a perfect choice. The village maiden might have conjured up Joe the blacksmith in her St Agnes vision, whom she might have dismissed while dreaming of great lords, but who would be loyal, loving and make her truly happy. Or if she or her family had been doubting a courtship, such a dream would enable subconscious wisdom to provide the missing clues and perhaps confirm the original choice.

The rites took place at times of the year when it was dark and cold and brought life and laughter. I consider them well worth reviving, if only to link us with the natural rhythms of the passing of the seasons that birds and animals instinctively know, but that we have forgotten in our urban cocoons. They work equally well for men and women – our male ancestors were probably just more covert about their romantic divinations. The rites offer too a reminder that if we trust our intuitive senses, rather than reducing love to a series of compatibility charts or spending night after night in singles' bars or clubs for the divorced, then there may be that special person waiting.

Practise the old love charms and you may see a vision of the one who is for you. The next day, when you meet for the first time in the supermarket queue or at work, you will experience the thrill of knowing that your astral souls were one step ahead.

If you are married or deeply committed and you dream of your partner on one of the sainted nights, you may recapture the first heady moments of love or passion. If you dream of another, examine your current relationship and perhaps face doubts that unresolved can lead to a slow death of love that might be revived with spells for passion and lasting love, and also take a cold hard look at expectations and practical obstacles to happiness.

And so the wheel is come full circle. Flower power and free love have given way to anonymous city apartments and suburbs where everyone retreats behind their front doors after work. The world can be a lonely place if you spend Sundays jogging round the park alone while the rest of the world seems to walk two by two.

But romance is not dead. In Durcal in Andalucia on Easter Sunday, young blades still serenade girls below their balconies. They hang a small laurel branch on the window of their beloved, meaning: *I want to see you*, a branch of orange blossom, asking: *Will you marry me?*, or if crossed in love the olive branch of peace, declaring: *I won't forget you*.

—— T W O ——

Attracting Love

W hen you are happy in yourself and with your-self, you are automatically more attractive to others. If you try the ritual on page 4 to raise your self-esteem, you may find that people compliment you on how radiant you are looking and the invitations start flowing. It is heady stuff and the more you believe in your inner beauty, the more charismatic your presence becomes.

If you are attracted to someone special or you have started a relationship that you would like to progress further or more speedily, however, specific rituals can direct loving, magnetic vibes towards the subject of your affections.

If you do not currently have a love relationship, I do believe that the cosmos will in time bring the right person your way by a process of synchronicity, or 'meaningful coin-cidence' as the psychologist Carl Gustav Jung called it. Nevertheless, you may wish to hasten the process as men and women have done throughout the ages, by sending out posi-tive vibes through attraction spells to someone with whom you would be happy and would make happy, if he or she wishes it.

Sometimes old rituals incorporate what seems, on first glance, to be dreadful doggerel. But remember the old skip-ping rhythms and playground chants from childhood.

Chances are you still recall them, because the rhythm and sheer repetitiveness etched them in your mind. It is the same with spells. Chants can be recited faster and faster as the spell energy builds up, or you can repeat a phrase as a mantra as you run your fingers through herbs, charging them with your intention, or mix salts for a love bath.

((

MAGIC OF THE CRESCENT MOON AND STARS

The crescent Moon and stars are the traditional friends of all who wish for love; when the Moon first appears in the sky on the crescent Moon, it provides the perfect setting to attract love. A Moon magic ritual of this kind needs little preparation or formal magical knowledge.

✦ Pile high symbols of abundance – jewellery, crystals, fruit and flowers – in a circle around three silver candles on a silver-coloured fireproof tray, to represent the three main phases of the Moon. The centre candle symbolises the Moon in all her fullness, being taller and larger than the other two.

✦ Light jasmine, incense of the Moon, and sit in the candle-light as it reflects on the gleaming jewellery and wish for your love to come. Really wish with all your heart, and most importantly *believe* your wish will come true; not easy if magic and promise has all too often been followed by disillusionment in your experience.

✦ For this ritual, suspend belief and fill a strip of golden paper with the word *love*, in spiral patterns, until there is no room left.

◆ Burn the paper in the left-hand smaller candle to represent the waxing Moon, and call love, or a lover if there is someone you desire, softly to you.

◆ Catch the ash from the paper in the fireproof tray and see whether, as it has fallen, it suggests an image of perhaps how or where you will find love (see the dream symbols on page 70 for suggestions of meanings). Allow your intuition to tell you the significance of the symbol or picture created.

◆ Leave the candles to burn out in a safe place.

◆ End your magic by going outdoors, and if there are any stars in the sky repeat the oldest love chant in the world as you wish for love on the first star you see:

Star light,
Star bright,
First star I see tonight
I wish I may,
I wish I might,
Find the love I seek tonight.

◆ Identify the star on a sky map and when you meet your lover you can show him or her the star that brought you together. If a star is not visible, wish anyway, knowing that like love it is really there, waiting to be revealed. Afterwards, consult your sky map and identify a star that was in the position in which you directed your wish.

☾

EVOKING CANDLE VISIONS OF LOVE

If you want to glimpse the one to whom you should direct your love, candle magic is again the simplest method of visualising a yet unidentified lover, he or she may even already be known to you, although not acknowledged in a romantic sense.

This process used to be called imagination; now the term is visualisation, but it is entirely spontaneous and natural within the human psyche. If you day-dreamed in childhood about a handsome prince or princess carrying you off to exotic lands, or as a young teenager pictured yourself living happily ever after with a pop star or a movie icon, you have already carried out this exercise many times. It forms an integral part of many love spells and divinatory processes.

✦ Begin at dawn on Friday, Venus's own day, or after dusk at her hour (see the list of magical hours on page 243) when you are quiet and relaxed.

✦ Light a tall pillar pink or purple candle, scented with rose or lavender, both divinatory fragrances of love, and look into the flame with half-closed eyes, asking to be shown the one who will make you happy.

✦ Do not try to force any images, but let them form either within or beyond the flame or initially in your mind's vision.

✦ The images may be very hazy at first, but as you work on your spells they will get clearer. When you identify a form, concentrate on bringing it into focus as you would with a camera lens, beginning with perhaps a particular feature – eyes, hair, or even a distinctive shirt or dress.

✦ When you have the whole person, let the voice speak in your mind's ear; however unlikely, the words you hear may be those he or she speaks when you first meet.

✦ If you do know the person, do not be surprised. Especially in second-time-around relationships, partners often come from existing social or work circles.

- After a few moments, blow or snuff out the candle quickly, blink, and as you open your eyes you will see the person quite three-dimensionally in the after-image.

- If you do recognise the person, do not be surprised if he or she telephones you in the days after the spell, or next time you meet comments that he or she was thinking of you at the time of the ritual.

- Repeat the process over a period of days and you may begin to visualise scenes of your developing relationship.

- If you see different people, it may be that you are not ready to settle down, but have many potential directions – and perhaps relationships – in your life that must be experienced before true love finally comes your way. For some, love that flowers later may be best of all.

- Practise casting the image into a mirror to amplify the energies.

As with all magic, what you send out, you get back threefold. So the intent of giving love to this as yet unknown person is the best emphasis for successful love rituals.

Calling Upon the Deities of Love

No love spell of old was complete without summoning up Venus or a classical god or goddess of love to aid the petitioner. In love attraction spells, the virgin or maiden love goddesses are usually invoked, rather than mother goddesses or married deities. Many modern spell-casters still follow the custom of invoking the ancient god forms, but it is a question of what feels right for you. If you do invoke a love god or goddess by name, find out all you can about him or her.

In pre-Christian times, good and evil were not clearly polarised, so that even a gentle maiden goddess might have done quite atrocious things to a love rival or unwelcome lover. Diana was not averse to having her hounds rip apart those she turned into stags. It is therefore a good idea to read about the deity to be sure that you are invoking the right aspect, and to build up an image in your mind of the positive qualities attached to the goddess as you see her.

You are not summoning up spirits or worshipping idols, you are concentrating the higher love energies, some might say in a projection of your more evolved self. Collect pictures of the chosen deity and perhaps buy a statuette. For classical deities, museum shops are an excellent source of such figures and the Internet has many full-colour images of famous paintings.

Below I have suggested those maiden goddesses that are often invoked when seeking lovers or love trysts. Often the same goddess will appear under different names and guises, as her worship was incorporated into different cultures. While some practitioners do use the ancient gods and goddesses in their love and fertility magic, I tend to prefer to dedicate rituals to generalised powers of goodness and light in the universe. I have supplied details of certain mythology books in the reading list at the back of the book so that you can explore this aspect of love and fertility magic more fully if you wish.

Aphrodite, Greek Goddess of love and beauty, is excellent for new and blossoming love. Her name means 'born from the foam' as, according to legend, she stepped fully formed from the sea. She may be invoked for the gentle attraction of new love as well as for sexuality (her name is the root of the word 'aphrodisiac'). As a result of her love affair with Zeus, the father of the Greek gods, she gave birth to Eros who tends to be evoked in association with sex rather than pure love magic. Aphrodite is especially potent in candle and mirror spells, and for love rituals involving the sea.

Artemis, twin sister of Apollo, the Greek Sun God, is Goddess of chastity, virginity, the hunt, the Moon, and nature. She also presides over childbirth, although a virgin goddess. Because of her connection with the hunt she is more active than Aphrodite in seeking love, or perhaps encouraging a reluctant lover of either sex and for winning love under difficult circumstances. She is perfect for outdoor love spells and for casting your love net wide to attract an as yet unknown lover.

Diana is the Roman counterpart of Artemis, and because of her strong association with the Moon in all its phases, is Goddess of fertility as well as love. Like Artemis, she is Goddess of the hunt and a virgin goddess, but can be invoked in her role as an earth goddess and as a protector of women in childbirth. Her beauty and hunting skills make her a perfect focus for the pursuit of love, especially from afar.

Hathor, the Ancient Egyptian Goddess of lovers and love itself, is said to bring husbands/wives to those who call on her, and is also a powerful fertility goddess and protector of women. Also worshipped as a sky goddess, Hathor is frequently shown wearing a sun disk held between the horns of a cow as a crown. She is also Goddess of joy, art, music and dance and was once entrusted with the sacred eye of Ra, the Sun God, through which she could see all things.

She carries a shield that reflects back all things in their true light and from which she fashioned the first magic mirror. One side was endowed with the power of Ra's eye to see everything, no matter how distant in miles or how far into the future. The other side showed the gazer in his or her true light and only a brave person could look at it without flinching.

She can therefore be invoked for all forms of mirror love magic and is also associated with gold and turquoise; jewellery made of these materials can be a focus for her powers. Because of her link with the Eye of Truth and also with harmony, the love she inspires is noble and dignified and she can be a good goddess under whose auspices to practise love divination if you are having doubts about the wisdom of beginning or continuing a relationship.

Venus, the Roman counterpart of Aphrodite, gave birth to Cupid as a result of her liaison with Mercury. Although she had many lovers, she is the Goddess of chastity in women and is a joy bringer, so represents not only sexual pleasure, but innocent love and especially love in the springtime. She is therefore the focus in all kinds of love rituals. Cupid has fallen out of favour in modern love spells, possibly because the still predominant Victorian image of a chubby infant armed with bow and arrow is not in keeping with modern tastes. However, as the Evening Star, Venus displays warrior qualities and so can also be invoked for courage in love and for strength against a cruel or faithless lover.

Calling Love in Candle Flames

As I have demonstrated, candles are essential in love magic, not least for calling an unknown or reluctant lover. Pins were also traditionally used in such spells to pierce the heart of a lover (not literally, of course). One might be pushed into the side of a candle which was then lit with the chant: *When this wax melts, so melts his/her heart.*

In times past, many a gentle maiden would call her lover to her side in a fairly ruthless manner by piercing the wick of a lighted candle with two intertwined pins, saying:

'Tis not these pins I wish to burn,
But my lover's heart to turn,
May he neither sleep nor rest,
Till he has granted my request.

The maiden would then watch the candle and if the pins remained in the wick after the candle had burned past the place in which they were inserted, the lover would appear at the door before the candle burned down. If the pins fell out, it was taken as an indication that the man was faithless. The secret, as the damsels discovered, was to make sure the pins were securely fixed about halfway down the candle. Men also used this spell, albeit more covertly.

A word of warning at this point: spells demanding that the subject of your affection should neither sleep nor rest, even if thoughts of him or her are keeping you awake, are close to the point of interfering with the free will of another. There are many ways you can use candles and pins without trespassing in this way; a gentler version of this spell involves piercing the wick as before, and saying:

'Tis not these pins I wish to burn,
But a willing heart to turn,
Though I do not speak your name,
I seek your love in candle flame.

((

MAGNET MAGIC

Spells to attract an unknown lover sometimes incorporate such words as:

From north or south, east or west,
Let him/her come who loves me best.

Spells involving magnets are remarkably easy and operate on the principle of sympathetic magic. You draw potential lovers, represented by pins, to yourself, the magnet. My favourite version uses a silver-coloured mirror and a heart-shaped pincushion or pink fabric heart. This spell should be carried out for six days during the waxing Moon period just before you go to bed, six being Venus's number.

✦ Scatter at random pins or tin tacks on a map of your present area and the surrounding ten-mile radius.

✦ As you do so, say six times:

As pins are drawn, like bee to flower,
I call my love to me this hour.

✦ On a table covered with a green cloth, place a circular silver mirror, the colour and metal of Diana and all Moon goddesses.

✦ Light small silver candles in a semi-circle around the mirror so that their glow is reflected in it.

✦ With a clockwise sweep with the magnet, starting from the north, pick up all your pins, repeating as you do so:

As pins are drawn, like moths to light,
Come love to me, come to my sight.

✦ When all the pins are on the magnet, place it on top of the heart in the centre of the mirror.

✦ Gaze down into the mirror in the candlelight, trying not to cast your own reflection in it, and you may be rewarded with a shadowy image of a potential lover in your mind's eye or in the right-hand corner of the mirror;

according to mirror magic lore, images in the right-hand corner represent people or events that are coming into your life.

✦ Blow out each of the candles in turn, repeating the gentle candle invocation:

Though I do not speak your name,
I seek your love in candle flame.

✦ Place the map on your window ledge. Cover the area where you live with the silver mirror, heart, magnet and pins and leave it there until the following evening.

✦ Repeat for five more days, using the visualisation process practised earlier in the chapter. Each evening the image in the mirror should become clearer.

✦ On the morning of the seventh day, place the heart, pins, magnet and the map in dark silk in a drawer. You should begin to dream of your lover and may meet him or her on the seventh day. It not, repeat the ritual each month for six days, extending the range of the map – after all, your lover may come from the next county, state, overseas, even another continent.

☽

A LODESTONE CANDLE RITUAL

This is a more powerful ritual which can be used if love is slow in coming or if you want to further a relationship.

Use a red candle, rather than the usual pink or green, because red is the colour associated with passion. It is also the colour of Mars, the ruler of lodestones, who, it is said, was one of Venus's lovers.

Ideally, you should use a candle with three wicks to be lit

on separate days. These multi-wick candles are sold in many garden centres and household stores, but if you cannot obtain one, you can relight the same candle three times.

Lodestones, pieces of naturally magnetic iron ore, have for thousands of years been attributed with magical powers and until about five hundred years ago were regarded as living spirits. Paired lodestones frequently play a role in spells to attract friendship, love and mutual fidelity and can be used either to attract a new, as yet unknown lover, or more commonly to draw someone closer whom you would like to know better. During the Middle Ages a lodestone would be set in a woman's wedding ring and another given to the groom.

They are readily available and inexpensive and can be bought by mail order. However, if you buy them personally from a selection at a New Age store you can choose two that are powerfully attracted to each other, like magnets. Some lovers give one to their intended in a red bag and keep the second themselves, using the stone to call their lover psychically. You can even buy male (pointed) and female (rounder) stones, but in practice it is a question of finding two that attract strongly.

Traditionally, lodestones are soaked in water on a Friday morning until noon, left in sunlight to dry, sprinkled with iron filings or magnetic sand and kept in a red bag when not in use.

In the following ritual you can either visualise a specific person or be open to an unknown but positive source of new love, as you hold the stone representing your lover. Do not be surprised if the person is someone you know already but have only seen as a friend or acquaintance. Lodestone rituals can also be used to encourage fidelity, although it may not be wise to compel another person to stay in a relationship unwillingly for you may thereby lock yourself into a destructive relationship.

+ Begin the spell three days before the Full Moon at the hour of Venus after dusk.

+ Place the lodestones about 60cm apart so that their attracting faces are towards each other on a circular fireproof tray. This can be iron- or steel-plated as both are metals of Mars, the male focus. Set a candle halfway between the two lodestones so that it stands slightly behind them, forming a sacred triangle which is a symbol of increase.

+ Light the first wick of the candle and pass the lodestone to the left of the candle then nine times clockwise around the flame, saying:

Lodestone of love, stand for me,
Call my love, o'er land and sea.

+ Return it to a position about 5cm closer to the second lodestone and pass the second lodestone nine times anti-clockwise round the candle, reciting:

Positive and negative, Sun and Moon,
Joined as one, come love soon.

+ Return that lodestone to a position about 5cm closer to the centre. Extinguish the first wick, sending the light to wherever your love may be, and leave the lodestones and candle in place.

+ On the second evening, light the second wick (if you have a three-wick candle, otherwise relight the same wick). Using a taper, light two sticks or cones of rose incense, the fragrance of Venus, and put one to the left of the first lodestone and the other to the right of the second.

+ Sprinkle a few grains of sea salt on the second lodestone and pass the incense six times clockwise round the lodestone, saying:

Salt of life, breath of air,
Come true love, my life to share.

Move the lodestone about 10cm towards the other.

✦ Sprinkle the first lodestone with salt and circle the rose incense six times clockwise, saying:

I draw you closer, love, each day,
Haste soon to me and with me stay.

Move this lodestone about 10cm nearer to the other. Blow out the candle, visualising the light as beams encircling your lover and gently drawing him or her closer. Leave the candle and lodestone in position.

✦ On the third evening at the hour of Venus, light the third wick and sprinkle the first lodestone with three drops of vanilla essence or essential oil, the oil and herb of Venus and a powerful oil for attracting love and ensuring fidelity, saying:

As you move closer I extend,
My hand to yours O, lover, friend.

Move your lodestone about 15cm nearer again.

✦ Take the second lodestone and sprinkle it with three drops of vanilla, saying:

So close you move, I hear your heart,
Now joined in love, may we not part.

Move the lodestone so that the two touch in front of the candle and say: *As the wax melts, so do our hearts melt and join as one.*

✦ Very gently tie a long piece of plaited pink and green wool in nine loose knots around the joined lodestones and leave the candle to burn out. Each morning at dawn untie a knot, saying:

Love of love, power fly free,
Bring my true love safe to me.

✦ Until your lover comes, carry both lodestones in a red bag, and as a relationship develops give the second lodestone to your lover as a gift in a twin red bag.

((

A FLOWER AND CANDLE RITUAL

This ritual can be used to increase love and trust in a relationship. It uses flowers as part of a candle spell (see 'The Plants of Love'), and I have found that it seems to work especially well in the early stages of a relationship, perhaps when you are beginning to trust again after a betrayal or setback.

Carry it out, like your candle magic, when you first see the Crescent Moon in the sky, about two days after the New Moon period begins. If the weather is cloudy, check your diary or the weather section of a newspaper for the exact day when the crescent will be visible.

✦ Use a small, wide pink candle for the gentler aspects of Venus. Place it in a shallow holder or directly on to a small circular flameproof tray so that wax can form on the tray.

✦ In front of the candle, but not on the tray, place a symbol of your love, perhaps a theatre or cinema ticket from a pleasurable outing or a souvenir from a place you visited together. Traditionally, spells such as this would demand an item of your lover's clothing, a lock of hair or even fingernail clippings, but these are far too potent for such a gentle ritual. Even an unwashed glass that your lover held to his or her lips is a sufficient link.

- ✦ Circle the symbol and unlit candle with pink or white rosebuds. Use silk if you cannot obtain the real thing, or other small pink and white flowers. Do not be afraid to make substitutions to what is indigenous to your region; spell materials are only suggestions.

- ✦ Using a thorn from a rose bush (leave it on the stem to avoid scratching yourself), draw two hearts side by side and almost touching about a third of the way down the candle, saying: *Come love in gentleness and fill my heart with joy.*

- ✦ Anoint the candle with rose-scented oil – you can buy prepared candle-anointing oils or use a tablespoon of virgin olive oil to which a drop or two of rose essential oil has been added. Rub your candle from the top to the centre with the oil, using only a very tiny amount, and upwards from the bottom to the centre, saying: *Flow, love flow, flow now to me.*

- ✦ Light your candle and, by its flickering light, create scenes in your mind of quiet pleasures shared by you and your love.

- ✦ When the candle melts, so effectively joining the hearts, call your love's name softly.

- ✦ Leave the candle to burn through while you sit in the candlelight listening to love music, especially any tunes in which you both take pleasure. Let the gentle pink waves envelop you and let images come and go of your relationship developing in slow stages. Try to keep your lover's image in your mind's vision.

- When the candle burns out, draw a heart entwined with your initials in the melted wax, cut it out with a white or pearl-handled knife, and wrap it in light or white silk, keeping it in a drawer and looking at it when you experience doubts.

- You can repeat this ritual every crescent Moon if you wish; replace the old heart with a new one and bury the old one beneath a fruit tree, ideally an apple tree, a symbol of love and fertility.

A MOTHER EARTH GROWTH RITUAL

Variations of this ritual to strengthen new love appear in many different cultures under many different guises. You will need to obtain a footprint of the person you want to love you more intensely; use a patch of wet earth outside your front door or scoop up the soil on a damp day on a walk. Though marigolds are often used, I find lavender more effective to plant in the soil as a symbol of growing love, as it is a herb of loving relationships, affection and reconciliation. Its wonderful fragrance evokes optimism and strengthens the spell each time you inhale it.

- Wait until you see the crescent Moon and go into the open air – spells are more potent if performed directly under the Moon and not through glass.

- Take a silver and a copper ring, for copper is the metal of Venus, and silver the Moon. Turn the rings over three times in the palm of your hand and say:

Ring of Venus, ring of the Moon
Bind us in love that we may soon
In love and joy, as you do grow
Lady Moon like increase show.

✦ In an earthenware flowerpot, anoint each ring with three drops of milk, a fertility symbol, and then plant them in the soil containing the footprint. Run the soil through your fingers as you cover the rings to charge it with power, saying:

Grow love, grow,
Like milk let feelings flow.

✦ Plant lavender that is already in bud, patting it down gently and saying: *Grow strong, grow true, that our love may likewise flourish.*

✦ Tend your lavender each day and as you water it, say: *Grow tall, grow free, that our love may enrich and never stifle each other.*

✦ If your plant does not flourish, it does not mean that the love will die. Repeat the ritual on the next crescent Moon. All love needs constant nurturing and that with slower beginnings can often be the most enduring.

The Plants of Love

And I will make thee beds of roses,
And a thousand fragrant posies
A cap of flowers and a kirtle
Embroidered all with leaves of myrtle.

'The Passionate Shepherd to his Love',
by CHRISTOPHER MARLOWE (1564–1593)

So many love rituals incorporate flowers and herbs that you could carry out love magic with little else. Flowers are both the language and the symbols of love: a single red rose is given as a token of fidelity, a yellow crocus is traditionally worn on St Valentine's Day by young lovers, while bouquets are offered at weddings or to mend a lover's quarrel. Lovers of old knew the meanings attached to each flower and herb and would send intricate messages to each other. Even the way a flower was held when it was offered and received was full of significance.

Many of these love tokens were not exotic blooms, but humble wild flowers which, when given in love, are just as precious as the most expensive hothouse blooms. For centuries flowers have expressed the joys and sorrows, the pledges and betrayals of love. 'Oh my love's like a red, red rose, that's newly sprung in June' proclaimed the Scottish poet Robert Burns; 'There's rosemary, that's for remembrance pray, you love remember' cried the abandoned Ophelia in Shakespeare's *Hamlet*. Flower language received an international boost after Paul Simon heard the folk singer Martin Carthy sing the old ballad, 'Are you going to Scarborough Fair? Parsley, sage, rosemary and thyme', and turned it into an international hit. The ballad speaks of the four herbs which are used in love divination and are associated with thoughts and memories. And in the seventies, the folk group Steeleye Span had a hit with their celebration of the old custom of wearing willow as a token of fidelity.

The goddesses of flowers are deities of joy; the tradition of the Roman Flora, whose Floralia was celebrated at the beginning of May, lives on in the Floral Dances in Cornwall. Her festival and that of Maia, Goddess of merriment after whom the month is named, evoked unbridled merrymaking and passion as the world burst into flower, the trees were heavy with blossom, and fragrance rose from the herbs in the fields and along the paths and lanes. Under their auspices, love still can blossom for each one of us.

We do not need to be taught how to love or make love if we can reconnect with the natural world and the life force that flows through it, letting our feelings flow and following our heart and instincts and not an instruction manual. For love is not confined to humans. Swans mate for life and may pine away with a broken heart if one dies, while gibbons in Sumatra and the Malay peninsula sing love songs to each other and will always remain faithful to their partner.

The Flowers and Herbs of Love

In the Treasury of Love at the back of the book are lists of correspondences – lists of the traditional meanings of flowers, herbs, incenses, oils and trees – that can be used for all kinds of natural magic spells, so you can adapt all rituals using the knowledge that our great-grandparents had at their fingertips, handed down to them by their parents in the unbroken oral tradition.

The Magic of Roses

Roses, Venus's own flowers, are perhaps the most potent in love spells. From the pink rosebud of first innocent attraction through the full red rose of passion and fidelity to the golden rose of mature love, they are central to love rituals of all kinds, for example burning rose incense or adding rose essential oil and rose petals to baths to attract love, cooking for a lover with rose water (which can be bought in delicatessens), or substituting essence of rose hip or rose hip syrup to arouse desire. The blood-red rose is a symbol of courage and endurance if a marriage or relationship runs into difficult times. You can also plant a rose on a special love anniversary or the birth of a child, red for a boy and white for a girl, and as it blooms each year be reminded of the feelings of that first moment when the infant entered the world.

A Six Rose Pathway of Love

One of the oldest floral spells, from the days when most love matches were found in the same village, involved a lover strewing five red roses along the pathway between the two houses and calling the loved one's name into a pure beeswax candle flame at dusk. Then, from a sixth rose, five red rose petals were burned in the flame, one after the other, while the lover chanted:

Burn a pathway to my door, five rose petals now are four.
Four to three in candle fire, bringing closer my desire.
Three to two, I burn the rose, love no hesitation shows.
Burn two to one, till there are none, the spell is done.
Come lover, come.

The sixth rose was then placed in a vase of water at an uncurtained window and the candle left to burn in a safe place where its light was cast on the rose. When the rose died, it was buried, and if the lover had not come, the ritual was repeated with six new roses.

This remains a potent spell for hesitant lovers or where there has been a misunderstanding, or even to attract a specific person whom you would like to be more than a friend. In modern times it is more difficult to make a rose pathway between homes because lovers tend to live further apart. However, you could strew the five red roses from your own front gate or lobby to your door, or on a map marking the two homes, with tiny dolls to represent each of you, scattering tiny roses. You can even use an underground station route map if you normally travel this way to see each other.

Other practitioners drop the first rose midway between the houses if the lovers live in the same area, the second a quarter of the way from their own home, the third at the end of their street, the fourth at the gate and the last at their front door. If you carry out this spell, remember to put a fireproof tray under your candle and holder to catch the burned petals.

Though roses are the traditional pathway, you can substitute forget-me-nots, rosemary, sage or thyme to remind an absent lover of your existence, or parsley if you wish to kindle passion; the plants rather than the dried herbs are best as these are infused with active life force. Remember to call your lover's name in the candle flame before burning the petals so that if another person picks up the rose, it will not attract him or her as it has been charged only for your lover.

(

MAKING HERBAL LOVE POPPETS OR DOLLS

Love poppets or dolls were sewn by young girls to represent a lover or would-be love; these dolls were then filled with love herbs such as lavender or rose petals and the girl would sleep with it under her pillow, kissing it night and morning and speaking the words of love she was too shy to say directly to her beloved. Married women whose menfolk were travelling far from home would create husband and wife poppets filled with protective love herbs – basil to prevent infidelity, vervain with its promise of truth at all times, yarrow, herb of enduring love, and mint to keep away all dangers. They would slip the female doll into the departing spouse's saddlebag or pack and keep the husband doll in a safe place until the husband's return, replacing the herbs if the absence was long. Again, the wife would speak words of love at bedtime and in the morning, and in some eastern European countries they would have a tiny dish of milk and honey to offer to the doll, so that by sympathetic magic the absent husband would not go hungry and thirsty. Others made tiny beds of rose petals or lavender so that the man would be ensured a soft fragrant bed.

In similar manner a woman who wanted a baby might create a small herb poppet filled with chamomile and fennel, herbs associated with infants, and would create a tiny bed, pillow and blanket. Flowers and herbs were traditionally collected on May Eve by girls who wanted a lover, and at midnight they would fill a poppet with them. Girls would conspire with sisters and friends to get a lock of the man's hair (preferably pubic), and attach this to the doll with nine scarlet ribbons, saying:

Nine times I bind my love with red,
Bring him now unto my bed.

On May morning at dawn, they would gather a flower touched with dew, lie in wait for the man to walk on earth and make a footprint, scoop it up and put it in a pot, then water it with the dew that was believed to be a powerful fertility enhancer. On May night at dusk they would sprinkle this over the doll, prick their finger with a pin, let the blood fall on the doll and then wrap the doll and the flower in a white linen cloth. This was then placed under their pillows until the petals died; kissing it every night they would call the errant lover until he returned.

Modern poppet rituals tend to avoid using hair, bodily fluids or other links with the desired person, to avoid an intrusion upon the free will. They also tend to tread warily over such ancient binding as: *May he love me until all the seas run dry* or *For ever and a day*. Sometimes it is the spell-caster who has a change of heart a month or a year later, so time limits are perhaps best avoided, except in general terms.

The dolls can be created in an appropriate colour, pink for new love or for a baby, green to attract or increase love, blue for an established relationship and for fidelity, red for passion and orange for fertility. A featureless poppet is just as effective as one with embroidered features and wool hair. The herbs and flowers will give the doll extra life and potency.

You can make poppets to represent yourself and a lover, or an unknown love yet to come into your life, but it is important to retain the element of free choice by asking that the person will see you through the eyes of love, if it is right for his or her – and for your – personal path.

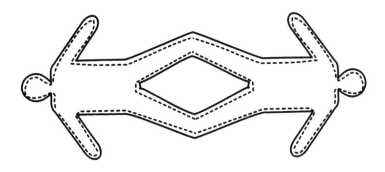

Pattern for a poppet: the dotted lines indicated where it should be stitched.

◆ Begin with your own poppet if you are making two. Just before sunset, cut out the number of shapes you will need (one or two) using the above pattern, endowing the figure/s with your hopes for the future and speaking words of love as you work.

◆ As you sew each doll, make wishes or name the qualities of your desired lover. Leave the head open to add the herbs.

◆ You can use the list of herbs and flowers in the Treasury to select the qualities that are important, for example lemon verbena for spiritual love, lilac for domestic bliss, mimosa for sensual love, mint for increasing passion, and vervain for bringing lovers together after a quarrel. Mix a small quantity to see how they blend. Add a few drops of essential oil to the herbs – lavender, geranium, ylang-ylang or neroli – to make your doll/s fragrant, or blend more pungent herbs with rose petals, lavender or other fragrant flowers from the list. You can also buy pot pourri flowers or blends; dried herbs or flowers are more concentrated and therefore better than fresh for poppets. (See 'Making a Pot Pourri of Love' below).

✦ When the poppet is ready, prepare your herbs or flowers, mixing them in a ceramic bowl or mortar, chanting – for example, as you make a protective doll: *Vanilla, vanilla, keep our love true.* As you place the herbs inside the doll, say: *May only love and light fill this image and bring an increase of love – if it is right to do so.*

✦ If you wish, insert a round rose quartz or moonstone heart on the left side of the poppet as you pack the doll.

✦ Finally, sew the feet, saying such words as: *Image sewn in love and hope, carry my thoughts to the one who will make me happy and I him/her.*

✦ As you cast off with nine knots, name them either according to the nine most important strengths of your relationship or a potential one, or say as follows:

Knot one for loving hearts,
Knot two for joyous moments,
Knot three for tenderness in sorrow,
Knot four for generosity,
Knot five for honest speaking,
Knot six for patience and forbearance,
Knot seven for laughter shared,
Knot eight for passion,
Knot nine that he/she will be mine as long as we both do wish it.

✦ Break off the thread with your teeth so as not to cut the bond with metal, or tie any loose thread in the final knot.

◆ If there are two dolls, bind them together face to face with red ribbon or thread tied in nine knots, saying:

Nine times with red my love I bind,
Joined in heart and soul and mind.

Place them next to your bed during the day and under your pillow at night.

◆ Keep the doll/s until your purpose is achieved or the herbs lose their fragrance, in which case you can refill the dolls or make new ones.

☾

Making a Pot Pourri of Love

Following the old custom, you can prepare batches of love herbs and flowers, not only for poppets but for filling love sachets or you can leave bowls of love herbs and flowers around the bedroom or in a bowl on your desk at work to attract and preserve love.

Either buy or pick your flowers and herbs just before dusk as the Moon begins to wane. As I mentioned in the last spell, if you are busy, you can buy ready-made pot pourri, or separate flowers already dried to blend into a mix containing the meanings you require. But there is something very soothing as well as empowering about seeing the whole process through from start to finish, and as you work you can endow each stage with the energies emanating from your emotions.

◆ Dry the leaves and flowers in a single layer on a piece of muslin, cheesecloth or similar porous material stretched over a large frame.

◆ Make separate areas in the frame or have a series of small frames for the different species as their drying times will vary. Place the frames in a warm dry area away from direct sunlight.

✦ Once dry put the different types of flowers and herbs in wide jars with lids. As you put each type in a jar, sprinkle the flowers with about half a teaspoon of salt each and orris root to preserve the flowers.

✦ When the jar is full, screw on the lid tightly and store in the dark for about three weeks. Label the jars with the date and type of flower/herb.

✦ Dry citrus peel in a low oven for about ten minutes to add to the mix for extra fragrance.

✦ Ideal flowers for love pot pourri include carnations, chamomile, cornflower, jasmine, heliotrope, honeysuckle, lavender, lily of the valley, pinks and roses. Because of their gentle nature, I have also used these very successfully for healing work. Suitable herb leaves include basil, lavender, lemon balm, marjoram, mint, rosemary, sage and thyme. You can also use pine needles and cedar wood twigs for psychic protection. Finally, suitable spices to add for potency and fertility include allspice, cinnamon, cloves, juniper berries and nutmeg, all of which contain natural energising powers.

✦ Either combine the herbs and flowers or make separate floral and herb fragrances. Good fixatives for their cohesive and preserving powers include powdered frankincense, myrrh, orris root, sandalwood or a few drops of clary sage or oregano essential oil.

✦ Experiment with the fragrance mix by combining a few petals or leaves of different species at a time, removing any that either overpower or clash with others.

✦ Use 3 cups of dried flowers and leaves to 2 tablespoons of powdered spice, 6 drops of an essential oil for extra fragrance, for example lavender, lemon, orange, neroli, geranium or rose, 1 tablespoon of fixing powder or up to 6 drops of the fixing oil.

✦ Mix the pot pourri ingredients together with a wooden spoon or your fingers and store them in sealed dark jars for a few weeks. As you work, say as a mantra:

Bound in love, but willingly, bound in thoughts, and dreams are we.
Dreams are many, hours are few; timeless though if love is true.
Bond heart to heart, you fragrant flowers, these herbs of love, our love empowers.

Making Herb Sachets for Love

Herb sachets can be pinned to an item of clothing or carried in a bag or pocket. They are very easy to make and at their simplest are no more than a piece of cloth or small porous bag in which the herbs are tied.

✦ Give the chosen herbs or pot pourri extra power by running them through your fingers into a ceramic or wooden bowl, repeating, for example: *Lavender, lavender, bring me love*, until you can feel their power rising.

✦ Use a square of about 10–25cm, depending on whether you want to wear the sachet or put it under your pillow, made of a natural fabric such as felt, wool or cotton, using the same colour associations as you did for poppets.

✦ Place about a tablespoon of dried, ground herbs and

flowers or the pot pourri mix in the centre of the cloth, using more for a larger sachet.

✦ Tie the material using three consecutive knots of a natural twine of the same colour as the bag, seeing your energy and hopes bound in the knots. As you tie your bag, visualise yourself and your true love after your wish has been realised.

✦ Carry the sachet until it loses its fragrance, or if the love matter will take many months to come to fruition replace the herbs regularly by opening the sachet and scattering some of the old herbs to the four winds, burning a few, burying some and dissolving the rest in water.

✦ Empower new herbs and refill the sachet.

A Venus Sachet for Attracting Love and Fidelity

If you are skilled at sewing you can make a heart-shaped sachet and place it beneath your pillow each night.

✦ Use 3 parts red or pink rose petals, 2 parts heather, 1 part elder flower, 1 part goldenseal, 1 part pennyroyal, 1 part vervain.

✦ Add 2 drops of lemon grass and 2 drops of geranium essential oil.

✦ Before you seal the heart, add a jade or rose quartz crystal.

The Language of Flowers

The idea of a 'language of flowers' was popularised in Victorian times, but dates back thousands of years. During the time of Elizabeth I in England, flower meanings appeared in verse and Shakespearean plays, for example gilliflowers as symbols of gentleness, cowslips of wise counsel, pansies for thoughts and marigolds for married love.

Bouquets containing floral messages were a safe and secret way of sending loving thoughts, a promise or offer, warning or instruction, even across language barriers. Many of the flowers can be found around the world but you can easily adapt the flora of your environment. White flowers often indicate innocence or secrecy; red, love or passion; and yellow, warnings or jealousy. Delicate colours indicate gentler emotions or wishes than brilliant hues. Spring flowers reflect new hopes, summer blooms high passion or fulfilled love, while autumn blooms speak of waning or gentler affections. A full-petalled flower represents an intense emotion while a small flower can indicate uncertainty. A tall flower talks of lofty ambitions or a spiritual desire while a flower close to the ground or folded can show affection, friendship or uncertainty.

There are many variations of flower meanings and sometimes the reasons for the associations have been lost. Those listed below combine several systems with fairly consistent meanings. If flowers have special meanings for you or someone close, use your own personal interpretation. It is quite possible to send floral messages using wild or garden flowers, blossom or even silk flowers.

Flower Meanings

Acacia 'I value our friendship very much.'

Almond Blossom 'Your attentions are displeasing to me.'

Anemones 'I hope to see you very soon.'

Apple Blossom 'You are both beautiful and worthy of respect.'

Azalea 'Be careful we are not seen together.'

Bee-orchid 'Forgive me. You misunderstood my words.'

Begonia 'We must hide our love. We are being watched.'

Bluebell 'I will be faithful to you.'

Broom/gorse 'My only aim is to make you happy.'

Bulrush 'Be more subtle in your approach.'

Buttercup 'All I own I will share with you.'

Camellia 'Be brave in adversity.'

Campion 'Meet me at dusk.'

Carnation (pink) 'Thank you for your token/message. It was welcome.'

Carnation (red) 'I must see you very soon. Your absence is too painful to bear.'

Carnation (striped) 'I cannot see you again.'

Carnation (white) 'I have fond feelings for you.'

Carnation (yellow) 'You have proved unworthy of my affection.'

Cherry Blossom 'May our love grow a little each day.'

Chrysanthemum (brown) 'Let us still be friends, even if love has faded.'

Chrysanthemum (red) 'I love and desire you.'

Chrysanthemum (yellow) 'My heart belongs to another.'

Chrysanthemum (white) 'I will never lie to you.'

Clover 'May luck and health shine on you.'

Cornflower 'I am vulnerable, so be gentle with my feelings.'

Crocus 'You make me feel young again.'

Cyclamen 'I will keep you from all harm.'

Daffodil 'I am sorry. Can we try again?'

Dahlia 'Your changing moods make me uncertain how to approach you.'

Daisy (double) 'Your love is reciprocated.'

Daisy (field) 'You are my first real love.'

Daisy (Michelmas) 'It is better we do not meet again.'

Dandelion 'The future is ours.'

Evening Primrose 'Your love is not for me alone.'

Ferns 'Meet me.'

Flax 'Thank you for your kindness.'

Forget-me-not 'Do not forget our love.'

Geranium (dark) 'I am sad.'

Geranium (pink) 'Please explain your intentions.'

Geranium (red) 'I choose you rather than any other.'

Grasses 'I accept the way things must be.'

Harebell 'I hope you may change your mind.'

Hibiscus 'Your gentle nature is matched only by your beauty.'

Hollyhock 'May our love bear fruit.'

Hollyhock (white) 'I want to succeed.'

Honeysuckle 'Accept this token of my love.'

Hyacinth 'I regret our separation.'

Hydrangea 'Why have you changed your mind?'

Iris 'I need to see you soon. I have a message I must give you.'

Jasmine (Africa) 'I see you in my dreams.'

Jasmine (Europe) 'I desire you night and day.'

Jasmine (India and Asia) 'Our dreams of being together will come true.'

Jasmine (US) 'We may be separated but we are together in my dreams.'

Jonquil 'Please answer my question.'

Lavender 'I love you too.'

Lilac 'You have awakened new emotions in me.'

Lily 'My love for you is spiritual.'

Lily of the valley 'I had to go away, but I will come back soon.'

Marigold 'Your jealousy is destroying our relationship.'

Mimosa 'I understand your feelings.'

Orange blossom 'I seek a permanent commitment.'

Orchid 'You will want for nothing with me.'

Pansies 'Remember the happy times we spent together.'

Passion flower 'We are twin souls.'

Peony 'Please forgive me for my insensitivity.'

Poppy 'Life will seem better tomorrow.'

Roses (as part of a bridal bouquet) 'Our love will last for ever.'

Rose (Carolina) 'Our liaison will arouse anger in others.'

Rose (pink) 'I am afraid to show my feelings.'

Rose (red) 'I love you with all my heart.'

Rose (white) 'Our love must remain a secret.'

Rose (wild) 'I love you from afar.'

Rose (yellow) 'I am jealous.'

Snapdragon 'You mean nothing to me now.'

Snowdrop 'At least we have each other.'

Star of Bethlehem 'Can we forget the harsh words we spoke?'

Sunflower 'You cannot buy my love.'

Tulip (mixed colours) 'Your eyes hold my soul.'

Tulip (red) 'I want to tell the world how much I love you.'

Tulip (yellow) 'Do you not care for me at all?'

Verbena 'You have cast a spell over me.'

Violet 'I will not betray your trust.'

Wallflower 'I will love you in sad times as well as happy ones.'

Ylang-Ylang 'I am intoxicated with joy.'

Using the Language of Flowers

You may wish to begin by sending a bunch of a single kind of flower, or even a single flower, for example daffodils (regrets) after a disagreement, or lily of the valley if you have to go away from a loved one. A single cyclamen bloom would promise, 'I will keep you from all harm', while an iris would convey, 'I need to see you soon.' At first you might enclose a small note reaffirming the sentiment of the particular flower, or telephone shortly after the flowers are received. After a while you can share the language with close friends and loved ones and even create a floral system of agreed meanings to fit with the local flora (useful if a relationship is a secret).

Alternatively, create a vase of flowers conveying what is it you wish to say to your love and, sitting in the sunlight, hold each in turn and softly speak the message. You do not need to send complicated messages; two or three different kinds of flowers can express a wealth of sentiment. It is better to buy the individual flowers yourself and make up your own bouquet, as florists may substitute different species or colours.

Even the most impoverished lovers can send messages. Daisies, dandelions and buttercups tied with twine can promise: 'You are my first love and your love is reciprocated, the future is ours and what I have is yours.'

Seasonal Variations

The modern world has helped the language of flowers. With the improvements in communications and hot-house growing, many flowers are available for longer than their usual seasons so it is possible to combine what are traditionally spring and summer or even autumn flowers to obtain tropical flowers all the year round, even in cooler climates. Lavender once grew mainly in mountainous regions around the Mediterranean but now appears naturally in almost all parts of the world.

Giving Flowers in Person

The way in which a flower is given can also convey a wealth of meaning. Roses are most commonly used for this purpose but any flower with a thorn or leaves attached can be used.

A single rose on a plain stem offered flower uppermost shows positive hopes and intentions. A rosebud surrounded by thorns and leaves, offered upright, conveys uncertainty as to whether love is returned. If the recipient inverts the rosebud and hands it back, he or she is equally uncertain but not entirely rejecting the overture. If, however, the recipient removes the thorns and returns the rosebud upright, he or she is saying that there is true feeling. However, if the leaves are removed and the thorns remain, there is no hope of the love progressing.

Secret Trysts

Even if there is no need for secrecy, it can be fun to pass messages to lovers of which no one else is aware, using pre-arranged floral symbols. The white rose is the sign of secrecy and confidentiality, so if you include a white rose the recipient knows that you want to keep the meeting quiet.

There are various ways of conveying time, but simplicity avoids possible mistakes. 'Meet me' or 'do not meet me' can be conveyed by either an iris or by a green fern or other long grass or rush on separate stems for counting. The first fern given is either upright or inverted according to whether the meeting will or will not take place. The rest of the ferns are upright and the total (including the first) should be counted to give the day. One fern means today, two means tomorrow, and so on through the days of the week.

Dreaming of Love

Place under your pillow a prayer book bound with scarlet and white ribbon and opened at the marriage service, with a sprig of myrtle on the page that says 'With this ring I thee wed'. You are promised a dream of your own wedding and will see the identity of the groom.

This ritual is best practised on a Wednesday or Saturday.

If a man places a piece of wood in a glass of water or small bowl before going to bed, he will dream of falling off a bridge into a river. Whoever rescues him will be his love.

A Hallowe'en love ritual

Walk upstairs backwards eating a piece of Christmas cake and place the crumbs beneath your pillow. You will dream of your true love.

These are a selection of traditional love charms whose origins are uncertain, because they have been handed down through an oral tradition. Dreams are not only the royal road to the unconscious, as Freud suggested, but the pathway trodden by lovers and would-be lovers over the centuries to the dream plane on which barriers of time and space do not operate. As well as divining a future love through numerous rituals such as those described above, partners have spoken of vivid dreams in which they have met on the astral or dream plane and shared past lives together or visited strange lands. In the morning they have independently reported startling similarities in their shared dreamscapes. Fanciful or true?

Though the mechanics of dreaming are well documented, the precise nature of dreams remains elusive; however, many researchers have concluded that the dream state is the realm in which true astral or out-of-body travel occurs, taking love out of the here and now to the realm of spirit.

Dream Incubation

One explanation for the prophetic dreams which divine a future love – and also a method of inducing shared dreams between existing partners – is the tradition of dream incubation. This is the instigation of focused, meaningful dreams by a series of ordered steps that lead from conscious awareness to a dream state where questions can be answered and future possibilities glimpsed. Traditional countryside dream spells offered in simple rituals at pre-ordained times of the year were a means of incubating significant dreams for a specific purpose, usually to identify a future partner. Over centuries the actions became endowed with the cumulative hopes of all who sought to divine future joys.

A similar mesmeric waking state to invoke visions of the etheric or spirit double of a future love was induced by rhythmically combing or brushing hair in front of a mirror and is a feature of many of the love divination rituals, some of which I describe in 'Love Divination'. The now largely forgotten habit of brushing hair one hundred times before bed slowed down the conscious mind and so made transition to sleep easier and also formed a prelude to dream incubation. A dressing table set with perfumed pomander, hand-mirror and brush were common even until the 1950s, and it was a great sorrow in my life that I did not possess one, though it may not have had the desired effect of turning me from a chubby urban schoolgirl into a fairy tale princess with blonde curls.

Dream incubation was first practised by the Ancient Egyptians and the Greeks, and Aesculapian temples in the Classical world were sited at sacred wells and springs. Aesculapius was a healer who lived during the eleventh century BC, and later became worshipped as a god. These shrines are dedicated to healing, and dreams were the principal vehicle for securing relief or cure of illness and sorrows of all kinds, including infertility and impotence.

Love also came under the auspices of these dream centres and for centuries country girls would visit holy wells in order to dream of a future husband. One recorded case is that of a Victorian servant girl in Selby, Yorkshire, who visited the Fairy's Pin Well, so named after the custom of dropping pins in the water as offerings originally to the goddess and later to the saint or spirit of the well. Many of the goddess wells that were not Christianised became known as faery wells, especially those with strong Celtic connections. The girl drank from the well, asking the faery of the well to bring her a dream of the man she would marry. As tradition demanded, she fell asleep by the well whereupon one of her suitors, dressed in wedding finery, brought her a wedding ring in her dream and she was taken to Elf-land for feasting and revelry with her new lover.

Incubating Your Dream to Resolve Relationship Questions

You may be less concerned with visiting faery realms to decide which of a string of suitors you will accept, and more with solving a dilemma involving a present relationship or with making decisions that will benefit you and your partner. Dream incubation is especially good if you are talking round in circles about an issue as the dream world can widen the scope of possibilities and often provide an inspirational solution.

The first stage of dream incubation is to concentrate on the key question. If you want to meet your lover on the dream plane to work on the issue together ask him or her to carry out the ritual at the same pre-arranged time, or if you are sharing a home you can carry out the pre-sleep rituals together.

But dream incubation works equally well if you prefer to be alone. Indeed, if a partner is sceptical or uncertain about unconscious realms, try working alone a few times until you are confident and after a few sessions you may find that the partner will report a powerful dream about being with you and even describe the landscape you saw in your dream.

✦ List in your mind feelings about and possible consequences of confronting an issue and summarise the whole issue in a few words or a short sentence that will form the kernel of the dream. Write this down on a piece of paper. If your lover is not present hold his or her photograph or a gift to you and evoke voice, fragrance, touch.

✦ Repeat the question or issue in your mind as a chant, gradually slowing the pace and breathing more quietly and slowly.

✦ Place the words or photograph beneath your pillow; for

maximum effect place it in a slit or pocket in a lavender or hops sleep pillow which can easily be bought or made.

✦ Create a ritual to connect the before and after dream-time. For example, some Hawaiian people drink half a glass of water as symbolic of entering the dream state, while making the dream request out loud, leaving the rest of the water nearby. On waking they say 'As I drink once more, I recall my dream.'

✦ As you fall asleep, repeat your question or your lover's name silently in your head as a chant, gradually slowing the pace and breathing slower and more quietly, until you are asleep.

✦ Some people hold the sleep pillow as they drift into sleep, placing it directly below their head as the last waking action.

✦ Your incubated dream may wake you in the night. Keep a pen and your dream notebook by your bed and as you wake, write down fragments of dream, emotions or phrases that come to you.

✦ At this stage, do not analyse your dream. Try to spend quiet minutes during the day and let the fragments rerun and take on significance quite spontaneously – you may recall an answer, an action, or a dream symbol may become instantly clear. I have listed a series of dream symbols relating to love at the end of this chapter. Even if you or your lover did not share a dream, talking about the dreams you had can open channels of meaningful communication.

✦ Do not incubate dreams more than once a week as it is a very intense process and dreams need time to work unhindered in translating their messages.

Love and Lucid Dreaming

Lucid dreaming can be defined as dreaming while knowing that you are dreaming. Lucidity usually begins in the midst of a dream, when the dreamer realises that the experience is not occurring in physical reality, but is a dream. However, once this mental clarity in the dream state is sufficiently developed, you can use this awareness that everything experienced in the dream is occurring in your mind, that there is no real danger, and that you are asleep in bed and will awaken shortly, to explore and to take control of your dreams. This can then lead to the desired stage of using them creatively, to talk to lovers, change negative scenarios and, by successful interactions in dreams, to increase your confidence to explore and develop love relationships in different ways, thus allowing you to make more positive interactions in the actual world. Once you can dream lucidly, meeting a lover on the astral plane becomes much easier and dream incubation also can become much more directed.

If you and your love both dream lucidly you can interact deeply and meaningfully in shared dreams, and as a result your actual and telepathic communication will increase in the everyday world. If everyday communication is difficult or you have to spend many nights apart, you can talk without fear in your dreams, and because each of you can control the interaction, conflicts can be resolved more easily, even if one or other of the lovers cannot fully recall the dream the next day. In dreams you can ask questions and receive true answers. You can also communicate over hundreds of miles, make love and share time in your pre-arranged dreamscape.

Encouraging Lucid Dreams

It may take months of patience before you fully interact with a lover in lucid dreams. But each shared recollection, however fleeting, opens doors of communication between you. If your lover is reluctant to experiment with lucid dreams, it is again a technique that you can practise alone very successfully, and by creating interactions with your lover on the dream plane, you will find that you are more relaxed and less confrontational in actual interactions.

✦ If you want to share a lucid dream with a lover, select a joint symbol and create a joint dreamscape. This can work wonders for an ailing sex life and take an active one to new heights.

✦ Before you go to sleep, concentrate on your intention to know that you are dreaming during your next significant dream.

✦ If working alone, visualise yourself in an exciting or emotive dream with a current or future lover, or even a past affair if it can realistically be revived. Even if it cannot, a lucid dream can help you to tie up loose ends by giving your dream a happy ending, although this may involve you moving on to another more exciting or fulfilling stage of life or relationship.

✦ Create a dream sign in this visualisation, something that would not easily happen in the everyday world, for example a talking animal, a brilliantly coloured flower or a sensation of flying.

✦ When this sign appears, say out loud, 'When this [symbol] appears, I know I am dreaming' and continue with the scenario.

+ Evoke the symbol two or three times in your fantasy, repeating each time, 'When this symbol appears, I recall that I am dreaming.'

Let yourself fall asleep, but keep your intention to know you are dreaming and your dream symbol in your thoughts, so that these are the last remaining things in your mind before falling asleep. If you do attempt a joint lucid dream, recalling fragments the following morning may re-create some of the joy of the experience. As with dream incubation, for fully restorative sleep you should only attempt induced dream intervention in any form once a week. If you are working with a partner, you tend to dream positively about each other, even in spontaneous dreams, and as the ability to dream lucidly becomes more automatic you can change any negative scenarios that occur in natural dreams.

Keeping a Love Dream Journal

Use a journal for any dream work; if you are entering a significant period in a relationship, experiencing troubled times, or are alone and want love, monitoring your dreams not only helps with dream incubation and lucid dreaming, where dream recall is important, but can help you to understand your own hidden feelings, desires and fears.

+ Date each entry, noting any significant events occurring in your life at the time of the dream. This is of help when you come to analyse your dreams and in identifying patterns and recurring images.

+ Give your dreams broad category titles, along with significant phrases or keywords, so that you can identify patterns of dreams and events. This forms a basis for establishing your own dream symbol system.

✦ Note the location of each dream, its significance to you and the emotions it creates. If it is set in a place from the past, it may have special significance to your present situation, perhaps a rerun of an old situation that needs resolution if you are to move forward.

✦ Also note any recurring images and their meanings for you.

The following dream symbols have sexual or emotional significance. Of course you will still dream about money, the past, the future, career, family, friends, and a whole host of different concerns, and these symbols can apply in more general senses (see my *Complete Guide to Psychic Development* (Piatkus, 1997) for more on dream symbols). Because dreams operate outside time/space parameters, they can be predictive, not in the sense of a fixed fate, but by indicating opportunities just over the horizon that become more likely if you heed the prompting of the dreams, for example to express feelings of love even at the risk of rejection, or to speak out or widen your horizons. These interpretations are only a basis for your own symbolism, and you can create your personal comprehensive list of symbols.

Love Dream Symbolism

Abandonment
If you are left alone, whether by a lover, an ex-partner, or perhaps by your parents if you are a child in the dream, you need to examine the feelings of insecurity around your present isolation or relationship. Are your fears real or rooted in the past? If you are doing the deserting, you may be

expressing a feeling of being stifled that you have perhaps not acknowledged before.

Actor
If you are acting in a play, you may feel overshadowed by a partner or a relation and need to express yourself more forcefully and make sure your positive attributes are acknowledged. If you forget your words, you may be worried about others discovering your inadequacies.

Assassin
If you are being stalked, you should seek to understand the identity of the enemy in your real life, maybe a love rival or a family member who is causing trouble, perhaps behind your back. If you are killing someone, there may be something in your past that you are anxious to forget.

Bees
Excellent if you want to conceive a baby, as bees are an archetypal symbol of the fertility aspect of the Mother Goddess. Bees also represent communication on family matters, presaging rich and harmonious relationships and maybe forthcoming pregnancies or marriages in the family that have yet to be announced, but which your psyche has picked up on at a very deep level. Watch out for a sharp-tongued matriarchal figure.

Blood
A symbol of energy, action, fertility, a free-flowing life force and health. Menstrual blood or bleeding from a cut can indicate a loss of something precious or a draining away of your energy – take action to prevent this. Blood shed in violence may indicate vital issues bubbling beneath the surface that need resolving.

Boats/Ferries

Travel, changes in circumstances or location, may indicate a need to spend time with a loved one away from your daily routine, or even to escape alone for a while. Missed ferries may indicate pressure and fear of the consequences of slowing down.

Body/Nakedness

If you are naked in a situation where your uncovered body gives you pride and pleasure, for example making love or swimming, the dream confirms that the real inner person is at one with the outer image and that you are not afraid to show what you really are or express your emotional and sexual inner needs. However, if you find yourself naked in a public place or at work and feel ashamed of your body, or are aware that a lover is critical of your body, your self-worth may have been dented and you are afraid to reveal what you really are, either physically or emotionally, for fear of ridicule or rejection. Remember: the problem may be with the partner or other people who have made you feel this way.

Bride/Groom/Weddings

Any wedding celebrations represent a deep commitment or a desire for a permanent relationship. The identity of the bride/groom may be a prediction of the person who would make you happy. If it is your wedding, whether you are married or not, you are anxious for a closer relationship with someone and assurance that the relationship will last. If you are a guest, you may feel that you are being disregarded in a relationship in favour of someone else.

Bull

An ancient symbol of male power, aggression and sexuality, and so may represent the unfolding of powerful sexual and procreative urges in both men and women. If you are being attacked by a bull, it may indicate a fear of being overwhelmed by one's own sexual or aggressive feelings and the need to allow these creative expression, rather than denying them.

Burglar

If your home is being burgled, you may feel that outsiders are intruding upon your private life or that an outsider poses a threat to an important relationship. These intruders may be close to home – relations, for example, whom you have distanced yourself from in the dream symbolism to make the hostile feelings more acceptable.

Butterfly

An archetypal symbol of rebirth and regeneration, perhaps the awakening of feelings and trust after betrayal that have not been recognised on a conscious level. Positively, it represents the need to enjoy present happiness without imposing conditions or worrying about tomorrow. A trapped, torn or dying butterfly can represent a holding on to a rapidly changing situation.

Cave

An archetypal symbol of the womb, representing gestation, pregnancy and birth, and so an excellent symbol for all who are seeking to have a child. It can also represent the hidden sexuality of a woman. If the cave if claustrophobic, a man may fear being absorbed by a powerful partner or his own mother.

Children

If you are the child you may want to shed some of your current responsibilities and be free again, or you may be finding yourself forced into the parenting role too often in a relationship. If you dream of a child and want to have one, you may be preparing the way to become a parent; it may even occur on the night you conceive. Some people believe that they are contacted by the essence or spirit of a future child. If you lose a child in your dream, whether your own or an unknown child, you may be anxious that you have taken on responsibilities you cannot handle in a relationship. If the child is wounded, it may indicate old emotional wounds that have not healed.

Demons/Devil
There may be hidden negativity in a relationship that needs to be released positively, or there may be guilt about a romantic or sexual temptation that if pursued might threaten an existing relationship. In either case, it is better to confront the demons in the daylight and make a rational decision rather than an impulsive one.

Dragons
An archetypal symbol, especially in oriental tradition, of life-giving sky power, and therefore associated with male potency and with passion. If the dragon is fire-breathing and destructive, power may be an issue in a relationship and needs to be balanced rather than expressed in violent outbursts. Sexual frustration may also be a problem.

Drowning
Drowning can suggest fears of being overwhelmed by emotions or an inability to cope at times when you are presenting a cheerful and competent face to the world. If a child is drowning, this represents a growing fear that you cannot protect a vulnerable partner or an actual child. Share your fears and responsibilities, if possible, with your partner or someone close.

Eating/Food

If pleasurable, for example enjoying a feast, it is a sign of feeling at ease with one's body and basic instincts; it represents all forms of sensual pleasure. If you feel guilty or others say you are eating too much, you may feel deprived of physical affection or sex in the real world. If you are paying for the food and do not have enough money, you may be trying to pay too highly for love or friendship.

Falling

One of the most universal dream symbols and scenarios, representing the letting go of inhibitions and opening the self to new experience, and so a good indication of sexuality. Fears of losing security and of letting go of control may be indicated if the fall ends in disaster; examine fears carefully as dreams can offer hidden signs of valid but unacknowledged worries.

Father

At its most positive, the father (whether your own or a father figure) represents stability and security in a relationship. However, a forbidding, stern father figure in a dream can suggest restrictions and prohibitions from the past that may be preventing you from doing what you want. If a present partner assumes this controlling role in your life, it may be time to assert yourself, not easy if your confidence has been undermined.

Floating

Represents sexual bliss and harmony; if floating with a partner, potential unity on many levels. Pregnant women frequently have floating dreams as they connect with their unborn child. If floating through total emptiness this can echo a sense of isolation and purposelessness.

Floods

You may feel trapped in a situation that you fear will engulf you. A relationship may be progressing too fast or you are suffering emotional blackmail. If the water is dammed you are perhaps keeping your emotions too tightly in check.

Flowers

Flowers, especially roses, are the ultimate symbol of love and romance, so walking through a garden of flowers, even alone, suggests that if you are not involved in a relationship you will soon find romance, as your psychic antennae are working overtime. Seek what is beautiful and do not settle for second best is another meaning of flower dreams. A bouquet suggests you may have a hidden admirer.

Flying

Another image associated with astral travel, lucid dreaming, sexual ecstasy and an empowering and spiritually releasing image. Flying like a bird or flying in a plane marks the widening of horizons and so it is a time to travel either alone if you are unattached, or with a lover. Fears of flying or of flying too fast and becoming dizzy and falling can indicate a terror of losing control emotionally or sexually, and of being forced along a path you do not wish to take.

Forest/Jungle

Another archetypal image found in myth and fairy tale alike is the terrain through which the hero/heroine must pass. A forest represents untamed nature and natural instincts, so if you are alone you may need to take your courage and perhaps make the first approach in a potential relationship, or take a step into the unknown in another aspect of your life. If you are trapped by brambles or a mass of branches, you may be feeling trapped by the anger or jealousy of a partner.

Fountain

Another symbol of the Mother Goddess and associated with fertility, virility, birth and with the free flowing of emotion. If the fountain has dried up, your relationship may need reviving or, if it has drained you of feeling, you may need to seek another source of inspiration.

Garden

This image can appear at fertile times as an indication of the right time for conception, and during early pregnancy. In love it indicates a balance between all aspects of the relationship and promises growth of fidelity and commitment. A barren or untended garden means that spiritual and emotional growth are being neglected, perhaps in favour of others' needs or demands.

God/Goddess

This suggests that you are striving for perfection and seeking ideal love which may lead to missed opportunities because you find it hard to accept a potential partner's failings. However, it can indicate that the desire to communicate and to be understood on the deepest level is not being met in present situations or relationships.

Giant

Another symbol from myth and fairy story, a giant can represent an overwhelming desire or obstacle either to love or in a relationship, often when outside influences are proving particularly intense. But the power of the giant really can move mountains; another male potency symbol.

Gypsy

A symbol of the need or desire to be free of unnecessary restrictions, either of a restricting relationship or, more positively, of burdens of home and property or work that stand in the way of leisure time together in a relationship. Family may be pushing you down a conventional path you do not wish to tread.

Harvest
Another fertility symbol, and an indication that a current relationship will develop if it is nurtured. For the unattached, recurrent dreams of harvest may suggest that love will come in the autumn, but that now is the time to begin new activities or widen your social circle.

Holidays
Holiday romances in dreams for the unattached may suggest that you are feeling frustrated by your current situation and should take every opportunity to visit new places and meet new people. Holiday dreams with a partner should be followed by a short break or a day away, as they can indicate that you are both pressurised by home or work and are losing sight of each other.

Horse
A power symbol whether you are the horse or rider, especially of male potency. A stampede of horses or a horse out of control dragging you, the rider, along, can suggest that you are afraid of the powerful emotions or sexuality that you are experiencing, or are being rushed into a sexual commitment before you are ready.

Incubus (male) or Saccubus (female)
Dreams in which you are crushed or attacked sexually by a demon of the opposite sex usually occur in later adolescence right through to the thirties and are more common in women. Such a dream may indicate a sense of powerlessness

and an awareness of the darker side of life rather than a spirit attack, although in recent years research has linked these with the concept of alien contact/abduction for the purpose of creating hybrid children. However, such dreams usually reflect unwelcome sexual pressures.

Infidelity

If you are enjoying an illicit relationship in a dream, it can be a simple fantasy fulfilment, especially if the dream lover is famous or exotic; you may be working through sexual inhibitions that, if removed, can lead to increased sexual pleasure within your regular relationship. If you are being betrayed or are feeling guilty about betraying your partner in the dream, there may be suppressed fears about the relationship and trust issues that may or may not be justified.

Jewellery

Being given jewellery in a dream may reveal a need to be more valued in a relationship, not necessarily in material terms, but perhaps through acknowledging a commitment in the eyes of the world. Giving jewellery may suggest you are ready for this stage, but are uncertain how the other party will react. Losing a wedding ring can reflect fears about losing a relationship, or if you feel relief in the dream, perhaps a desire to be less committed.

Key

This dream symbol can appear if you are about to embark on a sexual relationship, especially for the first time. The key to a home can express an underlying desire to settle down, which can be surprising if you always saw yourself as footloose and fancy free.

Knight

A knight in shining armour may mean that you are looking for a magical solution or ideal person to transform your life. However, if you ride off with the knight, you perhaps have someone in your immediate circle who, though less glamorous than your dream figure, will offer you warmth and reassurance if you let down your defences.

Lions/Tigers/Wild Animals

These represent power and instinctive survival energies where ambition or success take precedence, albeit temporarily, over relationship or domestic issues. They also reveal a fear of being overwhelmed by one's own negative feelings, anger and sexuality, especially in a situation where another person or structure is dominant; and of feeling in danger of losing one's own identify in the face of aggression.

Love/Lover

If you are not in love at present, this indicates that you are receptive to love and will soon meet someone who, given encouragement, could be a new love. You may find that one particular person features, literally the man or girl of your dreams. These dreams may be especially prevalent around the old festivals. If you dream of your present love or he/she dreams of you, there may be issues that you cannot talk about – try lucid dreaming techniques for a meeting on the astral plane. Dreams in which your lover is faithless may indicate that your relationship needs care and a little vigilance, while dreaming of a past love suggests that your present relationship is lacking in romance or passion.

Magician

For women, a magician represents a charismatic older or more powerful potential or actual lover to whom there is attached a sense of danger, perhaps of forbidden fruit. You may need to use your head as well as your heart to decide if the risks are worthwhile.

Magnet

Indicates a forceful attraction, either to a person or a particular course of action, that if acknowledged will bring happiness. A more negative interpretation is the feeling that you are being drawn against your will to a destructive or repetitive situation that may bring disaster.

Mask

If you are wearing the mask, you may feel afraid to show your true feelings, being uncertain of the intentions and responses of others, especially of a lover. If your lover is masked, you may fear deception or that he/she is keeping a part of themselves hidden; you may need to explore this fear if you are to be truly happy.

Maze

Represents an unknown path, perhaps entering a deep emotional or spiritual connection. To be lost in a maze or meet a monster mirrors fears of surrendering certainty and of confronting one's own destructive and baser instincts – or those of a partner whom you may have put on a pedestal.

Mirrors

Used in many love spells to reveal the identity of a lover, in dreams mirrors are concerned with reality and illusion and may appear when much has been promised in a relationship, but little has materialised. A broken mirror, or one that reflects hideous images, expresses fears that the real self has been distorted or has even disappeared; also the fear of ageing and loss of beauty.

Moon

A root archetype of feminine fertility and all aspects of love, the Moon appears in dreams at moments of change when the natural flow and cycles of life are most powerful; the promise is that by following rather than resisting natural cycles, fulfilment and harmony will be achieved.

Mother

Dreaming of your mother whether she is alive or dead indicates an instinctive need for reassurance and wise counsel. Women frequently dream of their mothers when they are planning a baby, are pregnant, or in the first months of becoming a new mother and so are striving to reconcile the role of mother with wife/lover. Often the dreams resolve old conflicts and so release a woman from feeling she is in the mother's shadow.

Obesity

Being very fat in a dream and revelling in it indicates a sense of contentment and joy in sensual pleasures or an awakening of sexual passion that engulfs the body. In a woman, a swollen stomach can reveal a desire to become pregnant that may have been buried during waking hours. Negative dream connotations suggest guilt about self-indulgence and asking or taking too much from life; also the fear of rejection by others, of being undeserving, and seeking protection from hurt or rejection.

Quarrel/Argument

Winning a quarrel with someone close in a dream can pre-empt the clearing of stagnation and past resentments that stand in the way of future love or happiness. Losing a quarrel or becoming desperately upset can indicate your own uncertainties about values or opinions you hold, or a desire to disagree with someone important to you but whose anger or disdain you fear incurring if you make a stand in the real world.

Rain

A powerful symbol of fertility and male potency in many cultures and ages, for example in the sacred sex rites of Kunapipi the Earth Goddess in Australian Aboriginal culture that heralds the monsoon season. Persistent rain, a deluge or rain spoiling an outdoor event suggests the dissipation of energy and fertility or being overwhelmed by the emotions of others or your own hidden sorrows.

Rainbow

The rainbow is an archetypal image of new beginnings, of joy after sorrow, as sunshine after rain. Said to be a lucky omen, it augurs the fulfilment of realistic dreams and wishes and reconciliation after a parting or quarrel.

Recurring Dreams

Any recurring dream indicates that you should listen or act on it, especially if it is a warning. The inner voice will often use recurring dreams if it is not being heard. If it is of a particular place, try to locate it as you may learn something there or meet someone who can help you; if unattached you may be drawn there at the same time as a new lover.

Royalty

Kings and queens, according to Freud, stand for the dreamer's parents or parent figures, while princes and princesses represent the dreamer. As love dreams they may indicate intergenerational conflicts or issues affecting your relationship. If you see yourself as royalty, older family members may be saying that a partner is not good enough for you. If the royalty are being condescending to you yet you long to be one of them, maybe in-laws or even a partner are making you feel inferior or excluded.

Sacrifice
Making a sacrifice at an altar is an ancient symbol of dedication and can herald the beginning of a deep sexual or emotional commitment, especially if the ceremony involves ritual sex. If you are an unwilling sacrifice, you may unconsciously feel that you have lost part of yourself or that your needs are secondary in the relationship. If you are uncommitted and the dream is positive you may be ready to settle down when the right person comes along.

Sex
This can be a wish fulfilment dream if you are not involved in a sexual relationship, or if your sex life is less than satisfactory in the real world. However, all sexual dreams, especially fantasy ones, can form the foundation for a rich and fulfilling sex life or for the release of sexual frustrations if alone. (See also *Infidelity*.)

Snake
Freudian icon of male sexuality and potency, the snake is an archetypal symbol of rebirth (and shedding the redundant), fertility and the mysteries of the Mother Goddess. If you are afraid of or are bitten by the snake, you may fear betrayal or conversely be facing temptations yourself; in either case, this should be acknowledged.

Stars
A timeless symbol of lovers and would-be lovers, stars can form part of an astral dream or represent a relationship, present or future, with a twin soul.

Sun

The Sun is a universal symbol of joy, fertility, pregnancy, babies and children in their most positive aspects. Above all it is a reminder to enjoy the present, every moment of a relationship or life as it is alone, without demanding certainties or always looking to the future.

Telephone

Represents important urgent communication, perhaps over a distance, or the need to express feelings or put right a misunderstanding. It can also indicate that a former lover or friend may get in touch, or an absent lover will declare love from afar.

Well

Like the fountain, an archetypal symbol of life, health and fertility, and the entrance to the womb of the Mother Goddess. You may need to heal the past emotional wounds of someone close or assume a nurturing role in a relationship, but this will be very fulfilling.

Wolf

A nurturing symbol of the family and those close to you; if the dream features a pack of wolves, loyalty in a lover is assured. Being attacked by a pack of wolves can indicate a sense of being torn apart by family or relationship conflicts, or having to go along with a way that seems alien or wrong to you.

Fidelity and Lasting Love

Love's not Time's fool, though rosy lips and cheeks
Within his bending sickle's compass come
Love alters not with his brief hours and weeks
But bears it out even to the edge of doom

WILLIAM SHAKESPEARE *Sonnet XVIII*

However happy a love match, it is hard not to question whether such joy and unity can really last for ever, or whether spiritual or physical ecstasy can be maintained. Rituals to preserve a powerful, permanent bond through the years can create a psychic and magical ring of mutual devotion, of which a wedding or fidelity ring is the outward symbol, and can be used regularly to affirm and renew original vows of fidelity and trust on the spiritual plane. This ritual bonding can be of special value if a marriage or relationship has hit a mundane or difficult patch, keeping away fears and anxieties that might otherwise take root, or possessiveness that will stem the natural flow of love with suspicion and resentment.

Yet you may have problems that make you actually doubt the bond, let alone want to strengthen it. You may, for example, discover that a partner is being unfaithful, whether emotionally or physically; a soul mate at work or an emotionally entwined ex-partner outside the marriage can be as dangerous to its stability as any tempter or temptress. Natural and quite justifiable emotions of anger and jealousy can inflame an already volatile situation and prevent you communicating your true feelings in a non-destructive way, and making a clear decision about whether you want the errant partner back.

If you yourself are involved in an affair and are uncertain as to the best course to take, making yourself the focus of the spells can clarify to whom you wish to remain faithful – or if you do not want to be bound to either partner.

A Magical Place for Two

A magical space, away from children, relations and friends, creates a separate time and place in which feelings can be explored and bonds renewed after a ritual (which can be as simple as lighting a joint candle from separate tapers). When couples are so busy that they rarely get time to eat together and communication is confined to the necessities of maintaining a home base, the real communication that brought you together often gets buried as well. If the only words you exchange in a week are about a leaking tap, problems with the neighbours and servicing the car, sensual massages are unlikely to seem more than another chore before you can sink into oblivion in your own corner of the marital bed.

Some couples make love after or as part of a ritual, and I have suggested in 'Sex Magic' that sexual ecstasy can be a very powerful vehicle for magical and spiritual desire. But it is also important to talk from the heart and soul about hopes, fears, dreams, disappointments and triumphs, or sit in silence in candlelight holding hands and letting the positive emotions flow between you in the light.

Create a special area of sanctuary for yourselves. You can set aside an area of your bedroom with candles, crystals and perhaps a god and goddess statue that seem to represent the male and female principles for you. In same sex relationships you still need the two foci. These figures can be gifts from one partner to another on betrothal or on a special holiday or outing.

A small chalet in the garden, an enclosed spot under trees or a spare room with a lock will also serve, and if you keep the place fresh with flowers and a few cushions to sit or lie on, it will become associated with cumulative loving energies. If the sanctuary is not the bedroom, you need to declare this a no-go area for the problems of others, for disputes and the demands of the world. If a partner cannot or does not want to co-operate, create the place anyway and work on strengthening the relationship symbolically; use the place for gentle, private conversations and tender love-making.

(

CLEARING THE AIR

If there is a continuing grievance between you and your partner – and in many long-term relationships there are issues on which there is serious disagreement, such as an interfering relation who cannot be abandoned or serious money problems – burn cedar or pine incense in your special place for both of these are cleansing fragrances.

◆ Take a fast-burning rose candle and mark on it two small notches about 3cm from the top each.

- Scatter a circle of salt around it in a clockwise direction to enclose any negative feelings.

- When you light your candle, allow your partner to speak uninterrupted about his or her negative feelings.

- Empty your mind of preconceptions and listen, for there may be grains of truth and sense. Ask your partner to avoid words of blame or any that will diminish your self-esteem. One strategy is to try to avoid the word 'you'.

- If you or your partner do not want to use all your candle time, sit quietly, touching hands if you feel able. See the negativity being consumed by the candle flame.

- When the candle is burned down to the first notch, it is your turn to speak, again without apportioning blame.

- When the second notch is reached, scoop up the salt in an anti-clockwise direction and sprinkle it in a bowl, adding pine or lemon essential oil for cleansing.

- Tip the salt away under flowing water, such as a tap, saying: *Anger, go, flow away, trouble us no more this day.*

- While you can mark the candle with two further notches and relight it next time you meet to unburden your grievances, some people prefer to dispose of the candle and use a fresh one.

- After the session, go for a walk or carry out some positive physical task such as gardening or redecorating together, but do not discuss the issue. If it returns to your mind, lock it in a mental box for your next candle time. Try to meet again later in the evening for a positive candle session, so that positivity can replace the anger you let out earlier. If this is not possible, burn rose oil at bedtime and spend at least a few minutes of pleasure listening to music or watching a television programme you both enjoy.

✦ If you must work alone, draw a large single notch about 5cm from the top of the candle and express your feelings out loud, but try to answer each grievance on your partner's behalf as though conducting his or her defence.

Fidelity

Whether a relationship has been officially cemented or is a strong love tie, there are many factors that can erode the bond, such as pressures of work, frequent absences of one or both partners, relations or friends who may interfere intentionally or otherwise, children, money and health worries. Once quarrels begin, it can be hard to recall the original reasons for love and couples drift apart; outsiders may offer sudden excitement and promises of perfect happiness unsullied by unpaid bills, blocked drains, teenage angst or teething infants. If you are married to a serial adulterer, you are probably better off without the pain, but sometimes the nicest people are tempted to throw away a secure but seemingly mundane life for a whirl over the rainbow, especially if he or she is hitting a mid-life crisis.

While modern love magic avoids more potent binding spells for errant lovers or the piercing of waxen images of the office femme fatale or hunk, you can adapt many of the old spells to incorporate free will, but you can also psychically remind a partner that he or she is spoken for and erect a warning sign to would-be predators.

Entwining Love – an Ivy Ritual for Fidelity

There are many versions of lovers' knot spells, and these knots, consisting of three cords tied with *twice seven knots*, would sometimes be given as a talisman to a departing lover. A very old love spell involved a girl taking a lover's necktie or handkerchief and joining it with her garter. She would then tie it to the bedpost, reciting:

Three times this lover's knot secure,
Firm be the knot, firm the love endure.

This was used not only to attract a chosen love, relying on stealth to obtain the lover's garment, but formed a binding spell while a lover was away.

In a similar ritual a strand of ivy, cut on the waxing Moon three days before Full Moon, would be bound round the garments; ivy was a symbol of faithful and permanent union and as a living knot was believed to keep the union secure. Sometimes the ivy would be attached to an oak twig, a symbol of endurance and permanence and also a male potency tree. The problem with ivy is that if it binds too tightly it can choke a tree or plant, rather than support and protect it, and so rather than binding with the ivy I prefer to use symbolic binding power and cast the leaves freely to come back willingly.

In a modern version, which you can use to keep any love match secure, you can buy a pot of trailing ivy with strong, long fronds, a plant associated with marriage and women, or pick a length of ivy from around an oak or ash tree.

✦ Take nine ivy leaves, fresh green ones if possible, starting at the top of the frond and taking leaves alternately from left to right, saying as you pick each one:

Ivy, ivy, I love you, keep my lover true,
Though I would not bind him/her,
I would our vows renew.

✦ If you have a wedding or betrothal ring surround this with your nine leaves, but you can use any ring to symbolise love without end, saying for each one:

Round and round the ring of truth,
Love in age, love in youth,
Love in sickness and in health,
Love in dearth and love in wealth.

✦ Take a bowl of water collected from rain that has not touched the ground or from a sacred spring.

✦ Add the leaves one at a time, saying for each one:

Flow free in trust and harmony,
Unbound but joining willingly,
It is by choice, you come to me,
And so we pledge fidelity.

✦ Swirl the water nine times clockwise and see which two leaves move closest together. In a gesture of trust, bind them very loosely with some of the ivy frond and cast them into flowing water, saying:

We need no bonds to tie,
The roots of love that in us lie.

✦ Bury the other seven leaves in the soil beneath growing ivy, or in the ivy plant pot, and water the soil with the water.

This ritual is also good for curbing jealousy in either party and for making a relationship less stifling while strengthening the underlying bond. If you cannot obtain ivy, you can substitute honeysuckle or vine, the former symbolising an offering of love and the latter pure joy.

Fidelity Herb Charms

Yarrow is a herb of enduring love, said to keep a couple together for at least seven years, and so given to newly weds and used in love charms. Married couples keep the herb in a special sachet and replace it just before the seven years is over, and continue to do so throughout married life; this can be made into a ceremony of renewal. Alternatively, hang a ring of dried yarrow over the marital bed and replace when necessary.

When a Loved One is Absent

Basil, rosemary and caraway seeds are used in old love charms to prevent infidelity by an absent partner or indeed to prevent someone from leaving you, given the free will proviso. People who don't really want to be/stay with you are usually going to make you repeatedly unhappy, so if you have doubts that are rooted in experience, be wary about binding an errant love psychologically or psychically – combine love divination and logic. If a faithful and loving partner is going away on a business conference, works regularly away from home, or is in an environment where office flirtations are common, however, a gentle herb spell will provide not bonds, but a safety net.

Of course you cannot sprinkle basil, caraway seeds or rosemary over a departing lover as many of the old recipes suggest, without exciting at least some curiosity, but if these herbs are added as ingredients to a farewell meal, he or she will absorb the magical energies. Alternatively, put a tiny herb sachet inside the lining of a suitcase or in the corner of a travel bag. I have even heard of people gluing the herbs to a partner's shoes (see 'The Plants of Love' for instructions on making herb sachets). Charge the sachet with a sprinkling of salt, waft bay or sage incense nine times around it, and incorporate an element of a green candle – you can drip wax on paper, cut out a heart shape from the mingled wax and paper and add to the sachet when cooled. Finally, add a few drops of lavender essential oil or rose water. As you do so, chant a variation of the attracting rhyme:

> *Earth, Air, Water, Fire,*
> *For me alone my love's desire.*
> *Fire, Water, Earth and Air,*
> *May he only for me care.*

Also sprinkle a circle of caraway seeds or basil around his or her bag and mobile phone before the parting and, if you want to be really sure of your partner, glue a couple of caraway seeds beneath the label of their pyjamas or night dress, if worn. Rosemary and marigold soap or cream are also efficacious as leaving presents.

((

HIS AND HERS UNITY CHARMS

To preserve love, the old customs say, break a laurel twig in half and each lover should keep half; silver hearts and other charms that split in two can be bought.

In cultures influenced by Africa, the lodestone that I suggested using in 'Attracting Love' can also help to maintain love and especially sexual attraction in absence. The fidelity lodestone is best as a gift. You can attach a charged lodestone to the belt or in a red bag for the pocket or purse where it will guard your interests.

If one or both of you travel regularly, you can recharge

your lodestones as a mutual act of love and trust to help avoid uncertainties that can creep in when one party does not phone when promised, or if when he or she does, you can hear noises of revelry in the background.

You will need a pair of lodestones that draw each other strongly and fit well together as a pair, as for attraction magic.

✦ Place your lodestones in a wooden bowl or on a chopping board kept for the purpose. If you are working with a partner, have two bowls and roll the other's stone in magnetic sand; alternatively, use iron filings. Some practitioners add dried lavender and yarrow.

✦ Roll them so that they join if you are working alone, or unite them on the chopping board when they are covered with sand, rolling the pair as one.

✦ As you move the stones, recite the Sir Philip Sidney sonnet quoted on page 1. This seems to have acquired magical significance, but you can substitute any love poem that has a personal meaning for you and a partner. You can change the gender in this and other poems as appropriate:

My true love hath my heart and I have his.
By just exchange, one for the other given.

✦ Sprinkle the lodestones with a few drops of essential oil, rose or geranium for fidelity, or with one of the special love oils available at New Age stores or by mail order, saying:

I hold his heart dear and mine he cannot miss,
There never was a better bargain driven.
His heart in me keeps me and him in one.

✦ Gently separate the lodestones, keeping as much magnetic sand on them as possible, and place one in each of two red bags saying:

My heart in him his thoughts and senses guide.
He loves my heart for once it was his own –
My true love has my heart and I have his.

◆ Tie your own bag, or both if you are working alone, with six knots in red twine, the colour of Frigg, the Northern Goddess of happily married husbands and wives. In earlier times, hairs from the couple would be attached to the lodestones or they would be rolled in semen or menstrual blood. As I have said before, I am not comfortable with such intimate magic, even with those you love, however you may choose to exchange hairs from your heads or, if you have a baby, divide a lock from the first cutting of hair, which should not take place until the baby is a year old. These can bind the individual lodestones, but only loosely.

◆ Exchange bags and keep them closed while you are apart. When you meet again, reunite the lodestones and leave them on a red piece of silk in your bedroom on the first night you are together. Keep them in a single large red bag until you need to use them again.

◆ If you are not able to exchange lodestones with your absent lover, bury theirs in the red bag in a plant pot, with a moss agate and jade for the growth of love and basil or rosemary seedlings planted on top.

Return What is Mine
If your partner is unfaithful, the other man or woman cannot entirely be blamed. Infidelity is a complex issue and can have roots in a marriage where communication is lost and the couple have moved in opposite directions, perhaps over many years. But there are men and women to whom breaking up marriages, especially where children are involved, is a

challenge. If you probe into the past of these real-life soap opera characters, there may be a whole series of broken relationships; once the 'only true love of their life' has given up home, family and sometimes their career for them, the conquest loses its excitement and the seducer moves on to the next quarry.

Whatever the reasons for your partner's desertion, if you curse or hex your love rival you are damaging your own karma, so waxen images and pins should definitely not be used. However, if you do want your partner back – and you may not – I am convinced that by the old magical laws of cause and effect, you are entitled to demand the return of a relationship that may have survived over many years and is perhaps cemented by the creation and care of children. This way you have a chance of sorting things out without the intervention of the third party, or at least parting with less bitterness if the underlying differences are too great. You can add the words 'if it is in our best interests that he/she returns' as a proviso, because it may be that the deserting partner is determined to pursue the new love regardless of hurt (see 'Ending Love').

The sea, with its powerful tides, has traditionally been invoked for the return of loved ones. In an ancient ritual a woman whose husband was travelling across the sea would collect sea water in a bottle, and when he was due to return she would cast it into the sea saying: *I return what is yours, return what is mine.*

Sea magic has proved potent for the return of all wanderers; as the original source of all life and shamans, the magical priest and priestesses common to all indigenous cultures dive symbolically beneath the sea to negotiate with the Sea Mother for the recovery of lost souls. Sea spells are usually dedicated to Sedna the Inuit Sea Mother, Ran the Viking Sea Goddess to whom gold coins were offered as tribute, or

Aphrodite, the Greek Goddess of love. Coins with holes are well worth hoarding for sea rituals; the best of all, the current Spanish twenty-five pesetas, will soon be out of circulation.

(

A THREE-DAY SEA RITUAL FOR THE RETURN OF AN ERRANT LOVER

✦ On the first day, go to a seashore or tidal estuary soon after dawn and on the incoming tide pick up a white or cream sea shell and some bladderwrack or any other seaweed. Engrave your partner's name on a stone and cast it into the sea, calling his or her name as you do so.

✦ If you cannot go to the seashore, buy powdered kelp and a large mother of pearl shell and steep the shell in sea salt and water and play a CD with the sound of the sea. Release a helium balloon, on which you have tied your partner's name written on turquoise paper, over any expanse of running water, calling him or her softly as the balloon rises into the air. Direct the balloon in your mind's vision towards the nearest ocean, be it ten or a thousand miles away.

✦ On the second day, begin with a solo clearing the air candle ritual to shed all bitterness within the circle of salt, and then wash the ill feelings away. Surround yourself with pillars of light and ask that only positive workings may be carried out in love and a spirit of reconciliation.

✦ Blow out the candle and send love to wherever your partner is, saying: *Let him/her come back to me if it is in our best interests that he/she returns.*

♦ Take the bladderwrack or kelp and make an infusion by leaving it to soak for ten minutes in a bucket of hot water; use a tide table to find out when high tide occurs at the nearest tidal water to your home. If you are using seaweed, keep it in a large sealed jar after you have strained the liquid.

♦ Begin work at high tide. Using a scrubbing brush and working in anti-clockwise circles, clean your doorsteps, front and back, and window ledges with the infusion, and also use it to mop any uncarpeted areas of your home or a yard, saying as you work:

Flower of the ocean, flower of the sea,
Send my loved one home to me.
Keep him/her from harm, keep him/her from danger,
Return him/her to me, held now by a stranger.

♦ On your sea shell, engrave, write or paint a circle as one unbroken line in a clockwise direction, enclosing two entwined figures to represent you and your partner, and also your joint initials in an unbroken pattern around the circle. Surround it with a circle of salt, and with four pure white candles at the main compass points; leave them in a safe place to burn away naturally.

♦ On the third day, again as early in the morning as possible, take your bladderwrack and shell to the nearest shore and at high tide cast the shell with the seaweed tied round it and a gold-coloured coin (if possible with a hole in it) wedged inside, on to the seventh wave, saying:

Goddess of the oceans and of the sea,
I return what is yours, send mine back to me.

♦ As you turn your back on the sea, say: *I welcome without recrimination if it is in our best interests that he/she returns.*

+ If you cannot go to a tidal water, dissolve some kelp powder in salt water and add the sea shell, casting them into any running source of water, even a tap in the garden that flows into a water butt.

+ On the day after the ritual ends try to establish friendly non-confrontational contact with your partner, remembering that guilt can make people say very cruel things. Protect yourself with light and carry out the self-esteem ritual described in the Introduction.

Handfasting

Handfasting is a popular marriage rite among Wiccans, a nature religion that sees all life as sacred. The traditional commitment is a 'year and a day', which is then renewed each year in a rededication ceremony. Other couples promise to remain together 'as long as love shall last' or the more Christianised 'till death us do part', and for those who believe in reincarnation 'throughout all lifetimes'.

Handfasting is named after the focal point of the rite in which hands are loosely joined by a cord or cords to symbolise the uniting of the two people, body, mind and soul. There are many variations of the cord ritual: two separate white cords knotted together and then used to bind both hands of the partners together; a long black cord loosely binding hands crossed over the chalice, tied in a figure of eight and the knot tightened as the cord is held above the heads of the couple. My own favourite is a single red cord binding the right hands of the couple, based on the old Romany tradition. I have used this in the following ritual as it can form part of the ceremony if a couple perform the rite alone, and it also allows the placing of rings on the left heart finger to seal the left-hand union. You can, however, adapt the cord ritual as feels appropriate: right hand to left; single cords that are joined only in the binding.

In the US, if either the priestess or priest is legally registered, handfasting is recognised as an official form of marriage. Most handfastings, however, are not legally binding, though they can now be added to a civil ceremony or held separately. Among non-Wiccans, this spiritual form of acknowledging a commitment can also be carried out either with friends, privately at home or in an open place.

The custom of handfasting dates back through many centuries in the form of woodland weddings, informal ceremonies carried out in fields and forests following the old pagan tradition, often because a girl was pregnant and priests would not officiate during Lent. These ceremonies, which continued until Victorian times alongside church ceremonies that might follow after the baby was born, were also popular around May Eve when couples would spend time in the woods, gathering hawthorn boughs and making love to fertilise the fields.

True Romany gypsies still use handfasting, though they may also hold an official civil ceremony. In one version, in the presence of witnesses, a gypsy couple clasp right hands which are then loosely tied with the man's neckerchief or sometimes a single red cord, and they pledge their love. A loaf of bread is broken and a drop of blood from both their thumbs dripped on each half. The bride and groom each eat the piece of bread coloured by the blood of the other. The rest of the bread is crumbled over their heads so that they will never want for food, and the couple then leave the festivities, having jumped over a broom to signify setting up home together. The following day the pair return to the camp, having consummated the wedding in the open air, to join the ongoing celebrations.

There are many beautiful handfasting ceremonies that can

be found in the Books of Shadows, Wiccan ceremonial books of ritual and natural lore, or on Wiccan information sites, both of which can be found on the Internet. In the Further Reading section on page 251 I have also suggested books that contain ceremonies that can be adapted for Wiccan and non-Wiccan use. The version I describe on page 103 can be used as a private ritual of dedication or with one or two friends or children.

Though a priest and priestess officiate at more formal ceremonies, you can carry out your own blessings, calling on the powers of light or goodness or any personal deities. You can also assign different roles in the ritual to friends or even children, and this is a way of uniting disparate family members who can take part rather than just watching the ceremony, perhaps sprinkling a circle of salt, offering the chalice or holding the rings. Parents or children of previous unions can offer the rings or tie the cord, and this is a wonderful way of creating harmony around the couple. Older people, mentors or parents may like to lead the ritual and speak words from the heart or introduce poetry or readings.

If the wrong tools are used, do not worry. This is not a formal magical rite, but a celebration of coming together in love. Any passing deity or benign spirit would surely smile at the efforts of a young child to tie Mummy's cord and offer extra blessings. Too many legalised ceremonies are marred because the best man forgets the rings or Aunty Jane is seated at the second and not the top table at the reception. Create a setting that is right for you and those who will attend; improvise, be flexible and enjoy every moment.

A private ceremony for just the two people involved can be of immense value if a couple cannot be married for legal reasons but wish to cement their union, especially if there is a great deal of external opposition to the match. It can also serve as an annual rededication for couples who are either legally joined or united in love, or after a marriage has hit a serious difficulty. You can, as many couples do, write your own ceremony, incorporating love poetry, biblical passages or wisdom from any culture. I have used the terms male/female to denote the separate roles, but single-sex ceremonies need make only minor adjustments.

((

A Private Handfasting Ceremony

✦ Before the ceremony begins, whether you are working indoors or in a garden or clearing, sweep the area in anti-clockwise circles of increasing size, using a traditional besom that is on sale at many garden centres. If the area is paved, wash over it with a lemon, rosemary or tea tree infusion to cleanse it. An old-fashioned mop or the besom can be used in anti-clockwise circles to remove negativity, and clockwise to endow protection. Use eight or nine drops of essential oil in a medium-sized bucket of warm water.

✦ Good days for handfasting include the three days around the Full Moon if it falls on a Friday, day of Venus and Frigg the Northern Goddess of marriage. June is tradi-tionally a good month since it is named after Juno, the Roman Goddess of marriage.

✦ You will need a circular table or tree stump with two pure white candles either side of the centre, the left-hand one to represent the god candle and the right the goddess.

✦ In front of the god candle place a long red cord and in front of the goddess candle two rings on white silk.

Between the two is set a small honey cake or tiny fresh-baked loaf, made by the bride, groom or one of the parents or older children.

✦ Some people place a purple candle between the god and goddess candle, which they light towards the end of the ceremony with two white tapers, from the goddess and god candles, to symbolise two flames joining in love as one in the new union.

✦ In the north of the table (either use a compass or create a symbolic north), place a dish of salt to the left for the Earth element and a large gold-coloured coin to its right.

✦ To the east, set a ceremonial incense such as frankincense or sandalwood to the left for the Air element and an athame or black-handled knife to its right. You can keep incense sticks in a deep, open fireproof container so that you can carry the lighted incense safely during the ritual.

✦ To the south, set a gold candle to the left for the Fire element and a wand to the right, using either a pointed clear quartz crystal or a thin wooden branch from an apple or hazel tree, both trees of fertility.

✦ To the west, for the Water element, place a dish of rain water that has not touched the ground as it was collected; if possible, add dew from roses (use an eye dropper to collect this), as dew is a symbol of fertility. To the right, set a goblet of pewter, silver or clear glass containing red wine or grape juice.

✦ In front of the altar, lie the besom with which you swept out the circle on the floor, having shaken it first a distance from the altar and sacred area to remove all negativity. In some older traditions the besom stands, bristles upright to offer protection. In earlier times magical tools and every-day artefacts were interchangeable in folk magic and are a powerful grounding device.

◆ Scatter a large circle of lavender, roses, cedar and pine needles to create an area of purity and love around the altar, which should be in the north or centre of the room or open space where the ceremony is held, allowing plenty of room for people to move within the circle.

◆ Move into the circle with your partner (and any others present).

◆ The female takes the salt and sprinkles a circle clockwise beyond the circle of flowers, saying: *Within this circle we are protected. So will I nourish our relationship with daily words and deeds of kindness.*

◆ The male takes the incense from the altar and walks clock-wise within the circle of flowers drawing a circle of smoke at waist-height, saying: *Within this circle we are protected. So will I always speak and act true in our relationship.*

◆ Both stand facing north saying:

Three times the circle shown,
Now as the Maiden,
Soon as the Mother,
Last the Wise Crone.

◆ This links the female with the unbroken tradition of maiden, mother and wise woman/crone, the Triple Goddess first worshipped before Neolithic times as the changing cycle of human existence. The crone does not have negative connotations but represents the third age of wisdom and experience. If you are older, you may wish to adapt the chant accordingly, especially if you are a mother, but anyone, male or female, young or old, can enter a new marriage at the maiden stage.

- ✦ The couple move to the north and hold the gold coin in their cupped hands, with the female hand covering the male, saying: *All our material goods we share willingly with no division into yours and mine or blame if times are hard.*

- ✦ They move to the east and hold the athame or knife with the male right hand covering the female's saying: *We cut the ties that bind us to past regrets, anger, resentments and to any bonds that conflict with the loyalties declared now to each other.*

- ✦ They move next to the south and hold the wand, the male left hand covering the female's saying: *So do we kindle the fires of love and passion, joy and inspiration in and through each other.*

- ✦ Finally they move to the west and drink in turn from the goblet, the female first, saying: *So do we pledge as we drink separately for the last time support in sickness and sorrow, forgiving failings and strengthening any weakening of intention or endeavour.*

- ✦ They move next to the rings and pass each other's rings through the candle flame, the man's first through the goddess and then the god candle, and then the same for the female. He says: *With this ring, I pledge total love, strength, loyalty and protection, dedicating my body, mind and spirit, throughout many lifetimes/as long as love shall last/till death do us part.* She says: *With this ring I also pledge total love, strength, loyalty and protection, throughout many lifetimes/as long as love shall last/till death do us part.* (You can vary the vows as you wish. I like the concept of both making identical vows, but that is just a personal preference.)

✦ The rings are placed on the left heart finger by the other.

✦ They then take the cord between them and pass it briefly through the goddess and then the god flame, so that it does not burn, but merely sparks, looping it afterwards and knotting it loosely over the right hands, saying: *So are we bound willingly heart to heart, body to body and soul to soul, as one, forsaking all others, promising to create a safe and loving home for ourselves and for any children we may bear/have already created either jointly or singly.* (If others are participating in the ceremony, the ring exchange sometimes follows the cord tying, but it is a matter of choice.)

✦ The couple return to the chalice and drink from it together, saying: *We drink now as man and wife/pledged partners. May we never thirst in body, mind or spirit so long as we are together.*

✦ Next, they eat the bread or cake, saying: *We eat now as man and wife/pledged partners. May we never hunger in body, mind or soul while we are together.*

✦ The couple bring the besom into the centre of the circle, place it on the ground parallel with the altar, and with hands joined jump over it, saying: *So will we work as one, sweeping away what is no longer part of our new life together.* As they jump they unfasten the cord, which is then burned in the golden candle or the third one.

✦ At this point, if there is a third candle between the god and goddess candles, it is lit with two tapers from the goddess and god candles (she lights from the god candle, he from the goddess candle), saying: *So two burn as one. We that are joined in love and the light of the universe, God/Goddess, let none put asunder.* The cord is then burned in this candle. (In some traditions the cords/cord are preserved and hung on the wall, being used for any rededication ceremonies and then fastened to the first child's cradle. But this again is a matter of choice.) If there are children from previous unions present they can add separate tapers to the new unity candle so that they do not feel excluded.

+ Finally, the couple uncast the circle three times anti-clockwise, beginning in the north, this time using the wand, saying:

Three times the circle shown,
Gone the Maiden,
Now the Mother,
Last, Wise Crone.

You can carry out the ceremony at any time of the day. If just the two of you are present, as you leave the circle of flowers throw a handful over the head of your partner to ensure that good things will shower upon you and fertility, whether physical or emotional, will be yours. If others are present they should throw rice as well as flowers, which represents fertility. In warmer countries, where the rice fell after a wedding it would sprout up, and it was said that a baby would follow for the couple by the time the next crop was ready. Hazelnuts are also traditionally thrown, and brides in eastern European countries would collect and place next to their breasts an appropriate number of nuts to represent the children they would like to have in the future. The rest of the day should be spent celebrating or making plans for the future, and, if possible, at night sleep under the stars or at least in a caravan or tent, Romany style.

──── S I X ────

The Fertility of the Earth

Whether you live at the top of a high-rise apartment block, in a modern suburb of uniform houses with pocket handkerchief lawns, in the depths of wild countryside, or near an ocean shore, the power of the earth rises as it always has. But we can too easily become disconnected from its natural rhythms in the technological world and through the increasing urbanisation and standardisation of peoples throughout the world. Few people now celebrate the old festivals of love and fertility except in a commercialised sense; the Spring Equinox, for example, has become largely reduced to chocolate eggs and film-wrapped buns.

The birth pill and modern contraception have freed women from unwanted pregnancies. But when a woman is thirty-five and her biological clock suddenly goes into overdrive, pregnancy may not automatically follow and anxiety can set in, which can inhibit fertility. When lovemaking is governed by the ovulation chart or worse still a minicomputer, male potency can in turn be affected, if he feels the pressure to deliver. Infertility and lack of potency are usually treated as disorders of the body (which they may be) or of the mind, to be stimulated with sexual gymnastics, fantasies or the new wonder-drug Viagra. Yet in cases where physiological causes are absent, the blockage in the spontaneous flow of procreative energies may have its root in an alienation of the spirit from the rocks, the ancient stones, soil, water and the rushing winds that once formed the backdrop for human procreation.

Sacred Sites of Love

Our ancestors would learn from their grandmothers and grandfathers the special places of energy where couples made love in order to conceive a child: an oak tree in the forest that may be hundreds of years old and covered with mistletoe, the ancient Druidic fertility plant, a huge chalk figure, a sacred rock painting or rock sculpture, a standing stone, a holy well at dawn, a cave sacred to the ancient Earth Mother.

Though this wisdom is no longer handed on through the generations so readily, we can rediscover these places of power, often within a short distance of our homes, even in urban areas, and by making love there connect with the natural fertility of the earth. Some are still famed for their fertility powers, but many others are just waiting to be rediscovered.

Making love outdoors in a place of great magical significance, for example on the flat stone that often lies at the base of a standing stone, or on an ancient barrow or hilltop burial mound, where earth and sky merge, connects with the potency of men and women who throughout the ages have mingled their energies with those of the fertile earth. These power centres are believed by some geomancers and dowsers to be places in which natural cosmic energy enters the earth at a point where there are underground water domes, where water rises vertically from deep in the earth. Cosmic energy, which forms ley lines at these points, is regarded in almost every culture as yang, positive and masculine, emanating from the sky, the power of the Sky Father. Water is yin, negative in the electrical sense, and female, flowing from the womb of the Earth Mother. At sites where these energies met and harmonised, such was the experience of spiritual and physical power and well-being that they were chosen as places of worship thousands of years ago and have retained their potency.

Chalk Earth Figures, Rock Paintings and Sculptures

The Cerne Abbas Giant
The Cerne Abbas Giant, located in Dorset in England, is a true fertility icon whose powers have been credited with many pregnancies. It is also a place where men can increase their virility by contagious magic – carved in the chalk hillside, he is 180 feet tall with a 27-foot erect phallus. The Giant may be more than two thousand years old, representing either the Fertility God Hercules, or a Celtic deity of fertility. Suggestions that the Giant was a focus for phallic worship are given credence by the fact that the rectangular enclosure known as the 'frying-pan' or 'ring', about 70 feet from the Giant, has been the site of a maypole since living memory. St Augustine is believed to have smashed a phallic stone on the site of the enclosure, but seems to have left the Giant untouched, possibly because it was the huge stone around which the fertility dances took place.

The Giant was cleaned every seven years on May Eve, the chief fertility festival of the agricultural and magical year, and in a variation on the May Eve festival described in the previous chapter, when young people would spend all night

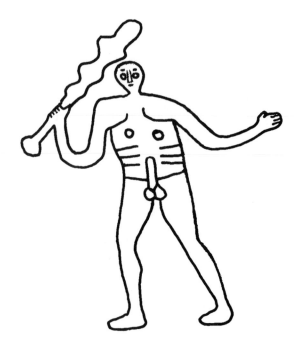

The Cerne Abbas Giant

gathering hawthorn boughs and make love at dawn in the fields to fertilise the crops, couples slept on the Giant so that they would conceive a child. Now the Giant is under the care of the National Trust and his maintenance is decided by official regulations which do not coincide with the magical seven-year ritual.

There are many attested pregnancies as a result of making love on the phallus of the Cerne Giant, and although the area is now fenced off, lovers remain undeterred. Andy and Sandy of Puddletown, Dorset, reported that after five years of trying to conceive they succeeded after making love on the Cerne Abbas Giant in August 1997, on the advice of white witch Kevin Carlyon. He told them to make love on the figure at

10pm on the night of the Full Moon while he carried out a twenty-minute ceremony on the Long Man of Wilmington, an ancient chalk figure of a slim human without breasts or genitals, sited at the end of the ley line that passes fifty miles across Kent, through Sussex and finally terminates in East Sussex.

The late Marquess of Bath and his second wife Virginia, whose ancestral home was the now famous Longleat House near Bath, a safari park as well as an historical monument, visited the ancient chalk giant at Cerne Abbas in Dorset in 1958. The Marquess and his wife had tried unsuccessfully for months to conceive a child, and like countless childless couples who spent the night on the hillside, visited the Giant with positive results. The Marchioness commented: 'I conceived soon afterwards and we call the child Sylvy Cerne in grateful thanks.'

There are more than fifty chalk figures in the UK and in the Further Reading section on page 251 I have suggested books that identify the sites of chalk figures and sacred places throughout the world. There are countless sacred rock or cave paintings, for example the Aboriginal phallic creator rainbow snake, Jarapiri, at Jukulta Cave in the Tanamai Desert in Australia, and rock sculptures, the latter natural formations that have, because of their shape, been endowed with the names and powers of deities or spirits. Around these the land is equally potent and since many of the rock sculptures are on high, inaccessible cliffs, you can lie and look up at them as you make love.

You will need to be incredibly discreet if you do want to make love on or near one of the ancient chalk figures or earth sculptures, especially as a visitor to ground sacred to an indigenous people. You may feel, however, that in the interests of ecology you do not want to risk damaging one of the ancient chalk figures by walking or lying on them, but anywhere in the area you are promised a truly magical experience. For example, the Cerne Abbas Giant can be clearly seen from a marked council lay-by about half a mile before the village, and as you look up at the mighty figure it is hard not to feel the fertility welling up in you.

To walk up to the Giant, go through Cerne village and up Abbey Street towards the ruined Abbey. Take a sharp right through the cemetery. There a sign will direct you to the old fertility and love well mentioned in 'The History of Love and Fertility', set in a grotto of trees and stones that form a circle; here you will experience the sensation of being enclosed within the womb of the Earth Mother, lulled by the gentle trickling of water and the blanket of green. Retracing your steps, climb over a stile on to the steep, open hillside and the territory of the Giant, the vast expanse of the Sky Father with all of Dorset spread beneath. The Giant is fenced in with barbed wire but you can walk across the hillside parallel to him and it is hard not to be swept up in the sheer power of wind and sky and the pulsating earth beneath your feet. Since it is difficult to make out the features so close, buy a postcard of the Giant in the village with which to identify the feet so that you can work out exactly where the most potent energies lie and make love on a direct parallel with the tip of the phallus. There is also a woodland to the left of the Giant or further up the hill.

You can gain even more privacy by staying in a hotel or guest house, or even a caravan or camping site as close to the figure, painting or sculpture as possible, having walked on or around the figure holding hands in the age-old tradition of lovers at midnight or dawn on the day of the Full Moon, the most potent day of the month. At Cerne Abbas itself are several lovely old inns and you could take back a little of the water from the fertility well to sprinkle on the bed before making love. Married women would also walk around the

Giant with their husbands before making love to ensure that their husbands remained faithful.

The rituals given in this chapter are entirely interchangeable and can be used at any earth figure, sacred site or holy well.

Creating Your Own Earth Figure

If you have sufficient space you can create your own fertility figure within which you can make love. Draw it so that it faces east and lie together within it at dawn so that you attract all the energies of the new day, create it in sand on the beach as the tide is coming in so that afterwards your cumulative energies are carried on the turning tide; etch it in the earth with a stick on a hilltop on the Summer Solstice, making love as the first light of this most powerful day breaks; use chalk in the back yard or patio at midnight, the transition of a new day, and surround it with pure white candles. The only limits are your ingenuity.

Alternatively, draw two outlines, yours and your lover's, so that they intersect like a cross; first chalk or crayon round your lover as he/she lies from north to south, making the outline about twice as large as the actual figure, then get him or her to draw around you in a different coloured chalk, lying across the first image from east to west. You can use wallpaper pasted together or large industrial rolls of paper. Make the figures intersect at the genitals and place the images under your mattress.

Stone Circles, Stone Medicine Wheels and Standing Stones

Folk tales abound of how, on May Eve, young maids would remove their undergarments and visit the Avebury Rings in Wiltshire to slide down the stones. They would then sit on a huge stone called the Devil's Chair and make a wish that they would marry their true loves. Circle dances around the old stones at these times stirred the fertility powers of the place, rising through the bodies of the dancers. If you allow your feet to move naturally around stone circles, single standing stones or ancient medicine wheels, especially in the spring and summer, you will find that you naturally follow a spiralling path.

One of the most famous fertility rings is the Rollright Stones in Oxfordshire. These stones are supposedly the remains of an invading king and his knights who were turned to stone in Celtic times by the legendary hag of Rollright. At midnight, a woman who wanted to become pregnant would go to the stones alone, remove all her clothes and press herself against the Kingstone so closely that her breasts and thighs were chilled. Within nine months she would bear a strong son. Such large pointed stones are associated with the potency of the ancient world tree of which the maypole is a relic and are still sometimes called 'tree stones'.

Making love on the flat stone of a monolith or single standing stone at dawn on a misty morning is one of the most spiritual and magical experiences, and if you call softly to the infant who would gladden your life, you may hear a soft murmuring on the breeze as his or her spirit draws near. In the Further Reading section on page 251 I have suggested a book that identifies many of the megaliths, the great stones throughout the world, but wherever we live there may be within easy travelling distance a single stone, usually unfenced in the middle of nowhere.

It is better to avoid Full Moon or festivals as these may coincide with local Wiccan celebrations at the site – or worse still the idly curious who expect to see werewolves and horned demons dancing around the stones. These stones are so powerful that you can visit them at any time to absorb the energies for they contain not only the impressions of those who created such sites five thousand years ago with only hand tools, but all those who have worshipped the Earth Mother in different forms for thousands of years at these sites.

☾

A Fertility Ritual at a Stone Circle of Standing Stones

This is a variation on a fertility ritual that I have given to people for some years and one which has enjoyed modest success. However, this version amplifies the basic spell by tuning into the earth energies, and it is an excellent way of uniting male and female energies in a symbolic conception rather than actually making love at the stones.

You will need to visit your stones or stone circle twice, once on the day on which the New Moon first appears in the sky as a crescent, and again on the day of the Full Moon. This is another ritual that you can carry out alone, but if you do carry it out with a partner, the male should hold the knife and the female the egg. A same-sex couple can modify the ritual accordingly, still using the knife and the egg.

✦ Take an agate or small hen's or quail's egg and a paper knife to the stones on the first day the Moon is visible. If the site is privately owned or a national monument you will have to adapt to its opening hours.

✦ The woman places the egg on a rounded stone or the altar stone. If there is only a single tall stone, use a nearby rock or the ground at the foot of the stone, having laid out a white cloth. If working on the ground you may find it easier to kneel or sit. Where I have not indicated who should speak, either or both of you can, as feels right.

✦ Surround the egg with a circle of white stones that you have found nearby, but not on the site itself, for sacred stones should never be removed from their source, saying:

In this egg is contained the potential for life, needing only the divine spark to give it form. I ask for the union of yang and yin, male and female, father and mother, sun and moon, sky and earth to meet here at this centre of sacred power within this circle of love, if it is right to be.

✦ The female sprinkles the egg with a few drops of milk, saying:

May this egg be nourished as it grows
so that the life within me may grow strong and healthy.

✦ The male should take the knife to the north and just outside the circle of white stones, hold it in front of him, raise it over his head and then bring it down to waist level, thrusting it towards the egg but not touching it, saying:

So does the light flow true,
penetrating all barriers,
to kindle the flame of life waiting within the sacred sphere.

✦ The male should repeat this at the other three main compass points, each time stopping short of the egg with the thrust.

✦ Wait silently for a while to absorb the earth energies and then wrap the egg and knife in silk and carry them home.

✦ In your bedroom, light a scarlet candle and place the egg and knife in front of it, saying: *Come inner fire and burn.*

✦ Prepare an incubator for your egg on the window ledge. You can buy a wooden or cardboard decorated egg in two halves or use the kind of pottery hen in which eggs are kept. If you have nothing suitable, use a small shiny silver wok with a lid or a silver serving dish also with a lid.

◆ Place the egg and knife not touching in the bottom half of the incubating egg and blow out the candle, saying: *Breath of life enter this new creation if it is right to do so.*

◆ Make love only if you wish to do so during the next few days, ignoring thermometers and calculations for this month. When you can tune into the urgency of making love and then experience an intensity unlike any you have known, that is the time when conception may most readily take place.

◆ Leave the uncovered dish or egg on your window ledge until the morning of the day of the Full Moon and then carefully rewrap the magic egg and knife in white silk for the return journey to the stones.

◆ This time, find a pointed stone or use the altar stone or ground. Again, put the egg in the centre but this time when you make a circle leave a gap in the east from whence new light and life will come.

◆ The male will take the knife and, beginning in the east, lift it above his head and then bring it down horizontally so that it gently touches and penetrates the surface of the egg, saying: *As we join in love so may we bear fruit of this sacred union.*

◆ The female steadies the egg and says:

So is the formless given form,
the potential moulded,
the unlimited brought within the confines of time and space.

◆ Take the egg and knife home and put them, now touching, in the large egg or dish. Light a gold and silver candle for the union of male and female, sun and moon, in a safe place in the bedroom and let them burn while you make love.

✦ Before you sleep, blow out the candles and send wishes for health and joy like the good fairies in the story to any baby you may have in the future.

✦ In the morning, wrap the egg and knife in white silk and place the second half of the egg or the lid over them until the end of the Moon cycle.

You can create a mini stone circle in your garden, following the pattern of an actual circle or creating your own design. This can be a focus for fertility rituals if you cannot visit a stone circle regularly and you wish to repeat the spell in subsequent months. It may take several months to restore the natural rhythms to your body, and sometimes it is necessary to wait until the time is ripe.

Fertility Wells

Sacred wells, regarded as the entrance to the womb of the Earth Mother, have always been a source of fertility for couples seeking to have a child. As Christianity spread, the former goddess wells were rededicated to Christian saints or to the Virgin Mary, who assumed the same responsibilities for healing and fertility and sometimes kept similar names and even feast days. The most common are wells now dedicated to St Brigit or Bride, the fifth-century Irish saint who shares a name and festival date with the Triple Goddess of the Celts: Brigit, Brigid or Brighde. The saint is also sometimes called the Mary of the Gael or the Second Mary and, as I mentioned in 'The History of Love and Fertility', was regarded as the midwife of Christ, who suckled the infant.

The Celtic Goddess Brigit would ritually mate with the

king or chieftain in the annual sacred marriage on her festival Brigantia, now St Bride's own day. St Brigit or Bride, whose animal like that of her Celtic namesake was the cow and whose attested miracles centred around milk and fire (the old goddess was the patron of smiths), became the patron saint of pregnant women, and to her prayers are still directed by women in labour and those who seek a child.

So too were sacred wells, both in pre-Christian and Christian times, associated with the breast of the Earth Mother, and on New Year's Day in Scotland the first to drink from a holy well is said to have the cream of the well and hence blessings throughout the year. The well of St Illtyd, near Swansea in Wales, is said to flow with milk rather than water at the Summer Solstice.

In age-old ceremonies barren women would walk sunwise around a pool or well three times, washing their abdomens in the healing waters, while the female keeper of the well chanted *eolas*, ancient magical songs, over the women's womb and breasts.

At the site of at least one Scottish well, a fertility ritual was practised into the nineteenth century under the tutelage of the keeper, in which women would dance clockwise in the cold water, first anointing their feet, then their breasts, and finally their genitals in total silence.

The Magic of Fertility Wells

Virtually all of the healing wells have specific rituals which, according to tradition, had to be performed in order to activate the power of the water. These can be discovered by visiting the local history section of the library in the nearest town to the well. Increasingly, old pamphlets of local folk lore are being reprinted as the originals come out of copyright, and these may offer clues. But if you cannot find any details of the old ceremonies, follow your feet, your hands and your heart. For we can know the old ways through our genes if we trust our innate wisdom.

May Day and Midsummer (June 24, but in earlier times the Summer Solstice or Longest Day itself) and Lughnassadh, the first harvest at the end of July, are days when well energies can be most easily felt. Since the ancient fertility festivals began at sunset before the actual day and lasted until sunset the day after, the period around the special days is also potent. Christianised wells were officially considered most powerful on the guardian saint's day or on Easter Sunday or Whit Sunday, but the earlier Celtic festivals continued to hold sway, especially for those asking for a child to be conceived.

The rite would generally begin just before sunrise and be completed before dawn. The well would be approached from the east or the direction of the rising sun, and the supplicant would walk round it sun-wise or *deosil*, a required number of times, either three for the Holy Trinity and Triple Goddess, or nine, an ancient mystical number of perfection. Offerings were invariably left for the spirit or deity of the well or spring. The origin of modern wishing wells lies in the Roman practice of casting coins in the waters to pay for healing or fertility.

Well dressing ceremonies in Derbyshire, Wales, Cornwall and parts of Ireland, date back to the early custom of leaving flowers as offerings, and flower petals, leaves, berries, moss, feathers, seeds and cones are pressed to form intricate pictures or patterns. Wealthier people would leave jewels, bronze or silver images of the healing deity, a baby's birth bracelet, or images of infants or mother and child in the waters. Many treasures have been discovered at the bottom of wells used in Celtic and Roman Britain and some of these offerings date back to the Bronze Age or even earlier.

A Wishing Well Fertility Ritual

You can make your own wishing well by creating sacred water and making offerings. For this, you will need to catch rain water in a large clear glass or crystal bowl. In Wales newborn babies were washed in rain water as it was believed it would help them to talk earlier.

✦ To remove any acidity from the atmosphere, gently drop a clear crystal quartz in the water, making a secret wish as you do so. Leave it in a bowl covered with fine mesh, if possible in a garden in the open air from dawn to dusk to absorb the life force or prana from the flowers and trees.

✦ At dusk, add an orange carnelian or a piece of amber alongside the crystal, making a secret wish for the as yet unconceived baby. Bring the bowl indoors, uncover it and surround it with tiny candles in pastel shades and leave them in a safe place to burn through.

✦ Just before dawn the next morning, standing in the east, walk around your bowl three times, and as you make a complete circle drop a small pure white flower in the water, saying:

Triple Brigid, three in one, bring to me a little one.
Triple Mother, sainted Bride, be a midwife at my side.
Triple Mother, one in three, give, I ask, a child to me.

✦ Light three pink floating candles in the form of flowers. Turn each nine times, saying:

Three times three, I offer fire,
Brigid, forge my heart's desire.

- Finally, sprinkle nine drops of milk in the water, saying:

  Mary of the Gaels I give,
  Milk that a new soul may live.

- Extinguish the candles as dawn breaks and, having removed the candles and crystals, tip the remaining liquid into flowing water, for example under a bath tap.

- If you have a water feature in your garden, drop a coin into it every day and make your secret wishes.

(

A Modern Day Potency Ritual

Magic is a tradition that has evolved over the centuries. Sometimes people perform rituals that have always been carried out at a certain place, imitating actions they have witnessed, perhaps without being aware that they are tapping into some ancient ceremony or unbroken tradition. Others go to a spot and find themselves behaving purely on instinct, in a way that people may have acted hundreds of years before.

At Alhama de Granada in Andalucia, Spain, there are thermal springs once used by the Romans and developed into hot baths by the Moors in the eleventh and twelfth centuries. The Moorish baths are now part of a hotel, but the locals go to the open springs down by the river, that spurt out of a hole forming a natural fountain in the rock and descend as pools of decreasing heat until the cold pool is created by the river itself.

Here I observed what seemed to be a modern-day potency and maybe virility ritual, although I was unable to ascertain its origins. Every few minutes youths would ride up on mopeds to the bridge spanning the river and strip down to pure white underpants. They would then soap their genitals under the fountain and wash themselves all over, before, still wet, pulling on their jeans and roaring off into the evening. My own observations were purely in the interests of research.

Love Divination

As a child, you may have plucked petals from a daisy or sent spores flying from a dandelion clock, reciting the old rhyme, 'He loves me he loves me not', little realising that you were tapping into an old love charm chanted by lovers over the centuries. Dandelions also act as transmitters of love; it is said that blowing the seeds from a ripened dandelion head in the direction of a lover will carry your thoughts, as well as answering questions concerning a lover's fidelity and intentions.

Will I find the right person? Will my present love last? Is he/she my true love? Which of two potential partners shall I choose? Should I marry or concentrate on my career? Can I leave my husband/wife and live with my lover? Is he/she faithful to me? None of these life-changing events can or should be decided on the basis of divination alone, for logic, common sense and emotions, as well as the effect of external factors and the intervention, welcome or otherwise, of other people, cannot be ignored. But if a solution is not clear or there are many conflicting issues, divination can give us answers using information not available to the conscious mind.

Because love is so central to the lives of so many people and is rooted in strong emotion, love divination has for hundreds of years been practised by lovers, borrowing the tools of their gardens and kitchens or consulting granny's tea leaves, rather than relying on more formal systems such as Tarot cards or astrological predictions made by professional practitioners. For this reason, love divination has kept a homely, almost earthy touch; as maidservants worked, they asked questions about their future happiness by scattering herbs plucked straight from the garden, planted vegetables named after lovers to see which grew strongest and fastest, or floated acorns in water to chart the progress of a new relationship.

How Love Divination Works

Naming a lover works on the same principle as all divination: the questioner selects by a seemingly random process letters or words which somehow give the name of the person that the deep unconscious says is or will be right for the questioner. The flash of insight comes from that area of wisdom where the barriers of past, present and future are not clearly defined, or, as others believe, from your guardian angel; these are not at all contradictory views. The methods can be incredibly simple or complex, as the following rituals suggest; try them with an open mind and with laughter and you may be surprised by the results. If you are happy with a partner, do not use rituals to find out who your true love is, unless you are having serious doubts. Even then you may be better scrying or using mirror divination.

Apple Love Divination

Apples have been connected with love and fertility in cultures such as the Celts, the Vikings and the Greeks and Romans, so such rituals are very old indeed.

Peel an apple and twist the peel once for each letter of the alphabet. The letter of the alphabet you have reached when the peel breaks is the initial of the first name of your future love. Others advocate throwing the peel over your right shoulder and seeing what letter it forms.

It is also said that lovers can discover whom they will marry by twisting the stalk of an apple and going through the alphabet, one letter for each twist. The letter reached when the stalk comes off is the initial of the first name of the spouse. To find the initial of the second name, tap the apple with the stalk, going through the alphabet once more until the stalk pierces the skin of the apple.

To find where this love will come from, flick an apple pip with thumb and forefinger while chanting:

Kernel come,
Kernel hop over my thumb
And tell me which way
My true love will come.
East, West, North or South
Kernel jump into my true love's mouth.

Where the pip lands indicates the direction from which your future love will come. If it remains static or flies up in the air and directly down, your love is very close to your present location. Some people flick the pips on to a map and then visit the town or even country on which the pip landed in the hope of finding true love.

((

THE BIBLE AND KEY

Traditionally, the ritual was performed at the turning of the year using a small Bible and your door key on a chain or string. In fact, the ritual can be practised at any transition time, whether personal or at dusk, midnight or dawn.

✦ Find the Song of Solomon, chapter 8, verses 6 and 7, and recite the words:

Set me as a seal upon thine heart, as a seal upon thine arm, for love is as strong as death.
Many waters cannot quench love, neither can floods drown it.
If a man would give all the substance of his house for love, he would be contented.

✦ Place the key at the appropriate section while you write the letters of the alphabet on pieces of paper or card, shuffle and place them face down in a circle at random.

✦ Remove the key, place the open Bible in the centre of the circle and tie the key on to a long red ribbon. Holding the ribbon with your wedding ring finger, walk around the circle in a clockwise direction. The key will swing on the chain.

✦ Continue walking round and round until the key remains still over one of the letters. The letter to which the key is pointing is the initial of the first name of your true love.

✦ To find the initial of the surname of your love, collect the letters once more, shuffle them and replace them face down in the circle. Recite the verses again, then hold the key over each letter in turn until it stops swinging. You will find that it stops quite definitely over one letter each time.

✦ Replace the key in the Bible, tie it with the ribbon and place it next to your bed. You will dream of your love and he or she will reveal their full name.

The Purpose of Love Divination

But can you really trust apple peel or a key to reveal such vital information? A few years ago I carried out the apple divination ritual on air with a well-known television presenter and the initials were not those of her husband. We laughed about old flames and secret admirers, but what I did not know was that her seemingly idyllic marriage was in trouble, though it was not until some years later that her husband's infidelity was revealed. However, I am also aware of people who have been given the names of future loves by clairvoyants and as a result an existing love match has been soured or potential relationships shunned because the lover has a different name from the one predicted.

Just as by some process of telekinesis – the power of the mind to influence inanimate objects – we seem to be able to select, for example, the correct Tarot cards to answer a specific question, so these old, natural forms of divination reflect the knowledge that comes from deep within us that is not constrained by time and space as the more conscious thought processes are. What these old predictive charms do offer is not a set-in-stone prophecy, but insight into the complex, multi-levelled web of past experience, present events and potentials, and so may alert us to some factor in a relationship that needs consideration, using logic and common sense as well as emotions.

The predictions do not usually refer to a love ten years hence, or a man or woman from the other side of the world, unless you intend to travel there in the near future, but someone who is around you at present in some capacity, a friend of a friend or a colleague at work. If, for example, the name Owen Richards or the initials O R appear in divination and you know an Owen Richards who works in Accounts, but to whom you have never spoken because you are lusting after James Moody who lives with his girlfriend in the next flat, maybe your subconscious is giving you a nudge in the right direction. Even if you subscribe to the twin soul theory – that we all have one man or woman to whom we are linked at the deepest level – there are a number of people with whom we could be very happy given effort on both sides. Sometimes it is a question of recognising such a person, or of moving closer to reality, rather than waiting in vain for the dream lover.

Equally, if you carry out one of the old fidelity rituals, a variation of he/she loves me/not, you may be asking an unvoiced question: can I trust this person not only now, but in the future?

To Find if a Love is True

A traditional method of testing fidelity involves throwing apple pips on to a fire while chanting:

If you love me, pop and fly
If you hate me, lay and die.

A loved one is named. If the pip bursts open with a crack, it is proof of love. If it burns quietly, there is no real affection on the part of the named person.

Of course, you should not divorce a spouse on the say-so of an apple spell. But if the pip does not crack, it may reflect an underlying worry that you need to resolve, whether the problem resides in your own insecurity – maybe a previous partner betrayed you – or if your lover's flirtatiousness is a problem and you are wondering about committing further or perhaps starting a family.

Options: Which One Should I Marry/ Should I Marry At All/Should I Speak Out or Remain Silent?

These option spells require time to come to fruition, very much at odds with the modern instant decision-making processes; if you do have a decision to make and the way is not clear, these spells can give you the space to let a love matter lie fallow and be revealed in its own good time. By consigning your choices temporarily to Mother Earth, the deeper workings of your psyche can likewise sift through the known and unknown factors. As you tend your plants, so you endow each with different aspirations and emotions, and few people now doubt what our ancestors knew instinctively: that our thoughts do affect plant growth.

Although our ancestors mainly used these methods for choosing between suitors, you can easily adapt them to help you decide between options, for example planting the number of onions or carrots to represent your different options in a decision to do with love.

Seed and Plant Divination

Onions

The most common form of love divination was for a young girl to scratch the name of several suitors on separate onions and put the onions in a warm place. The first to sprout would be her true love. You can also scratch a symbol or the initials of a decision that can take several courses, endowing each with the emotions resulting from the following that particular path. Once you have set up your choices, avoid thinking about them and let your unconscious mind do the work.

Carrots

This is a less pungent vegetable that works equally well. Cut off the end of two or more carrots, either to choose between potential suitors or to make love decisions, for example one carrot top for yes and the other for no, one for go and the other for stay, one for declaring love and the other for holding back. You may wish to write the names or the decisions to be made on paper and leave them under each choice.

Place your carrot tops on saucers and add just a little water when the carrots become dry (too much will cause the carrot to become mouldy). Leave them in a warm place. See which carrot sprouts first and that will give you the answer. You should have to wait only a few days. Use this time not to think about the love decision or the people, but to make your present world more fulfilling.

Mustard and Cress

Mustard and cress seeds planted on two or more saucers on either cotton wool or damp tissue are an even faster method of divination. Scatter your seeds generously on the saucers representing the alternative people or love choices. As you do this, visualise the person or decision involved in each and endow it with positive feelings. If the seeds become dry, water them gently, seeing the water giving life to your future possibilities and happiness. If you are asking about two people rather than a yes/no, act/wait decision, you can scatter the seeds in the shape of the initials of the people concerned.

Flower Divination

Flower divination is more subtle, as by monitoring the nature of the growth of each flower, you can follow the course of each option. Place two or more identical rosebuds, one for each choice, in separate identical vases and observe which unfolds first. This may indicate the best short-term option, but continue to tend the blooms and see which lasts the longest, this may be the best if not the easiest decision over a period of time. Did one have a sudden spurt of growth and stay fresh longer, before dying quickly? Flower divination works best if you gently stroke the stems, while speaking aloud your feelings about each option and repeating this each day when you water the buds. If it is a long-term issue, use seedlings of lavender, sage or rosemary and chart the progress of each hope over a period of weeks.

For example, Gina planted two seedlings to try to divine whether her lover Tony would leave his wife in three months' time as he had promised or if this was yet another prevarication. The seedlings both grew steadily at first, though she paid special attention to the one promising her lover would come to her. However, as the three months drew to a close, the plant representing their new life together began to wither. Though she hoped this was just a coincidence, when Tony began to make more excuses, she told him to go – and felt she had been prepared for this moment.

Anna's Flower Options

Anna is in her fifties and has been divorced for ten years. She met Nick, a widower, while she was on holiday in South Africa and they enjoyed an intense relationship. When she returned home, they exchanged letters which were loving on both sides, but Nick did not suggest their meeting again. Should she go to South Africa and risk rebuff or wait to see if he suggests that either he comes to England or she goes out there again?

Anna chose two pink rosebuds, which in the language of flowers means 'I am afraid to show my love'. One she designated wait, the other to go to South Africa. Before putting each in water she held them and stroked the petals, envisaging the positive aspects of both paths.

Each morning she added a little water, and as she touched the flowers continued the separate scenarios in her mind: the pleasure of receiving lovely letters and getting on with her very rich life in England, or catching the plane, arriving in the brilliant sunshine and being embraced . . . this scenario she could not seem to develop further at this stage.

The 'go to South Africa' option flower bloomed first. But Anna was not convinced. Going to South Africa might initially provoke a response, but would the relationship last or should she be content with the long-distance friendship and the possibility that one day Nick would invite her or turn up at her door?

Anna continued to tend the flowers and as she looked at the South African option, scenes of the developing love came unbidden. Wishful thinking? The 'go to South Africa' option continued to bloom long after the other rose had wilted. As an omen, Nick sent Anna a bouquet of yellow roses by international mail order – and so she has booked her ticket. Of course, she did not base her decision entirely on flower options, but the results confirmed what she felt deep down but was afraid to acknowledge: that if she did not go she might regret it all her life.

Love Divination in Water to Chart the Progress of a Relationship

Place two acorns in a large bowl of water. Designate one for each of you.

✦ If they float instantly close, the relationship will develop rapidly. If your partnership is long-standing, you are close on a very deep level.

◆ If the acorns float completely separately or in opposite directions, perhaps you have an unresolved worry you need to share or are not ready for a deep commitment in your present relationship. Go slowly.

◆ If your acorns float close and then away and back again, your relationship is full of the normal ups and downs but perhaps needs more romantic input to rekindle the flames of passion.

◆ If only one acorn moves, then that person is making all the efforts – is it worth pursuing such a course indefinitely?

◆ If neither acorn moves, then either there is no real attraction or there is a major sticking point that has locked you both in an intractable position.

You can add other acorns for those who influence your relationship – in-laws, children, partners – and the movement between all the acorns can be very revealing. Look especially at the acorn that stands between you and your lover – it may not be who you think, or one partner may be colluding albeit unconsciously in the conflict. Some people can hold terrific power if they have a partner and a parent competing for their attention.

Should your lover be absent or estranged but the divination suggests you still have underlying trust or optimism, pick two acorns with oak leaves attached. Wrap these in ash leaves on which the seeds or keys are still attached. Place them under your pillow, saying 'Acorn cup and ashen key, bring my true love safe to me.'

If you cannot obtain acorns, use corks, preferably from bottles used at a love or family celebration.

Mirror Divination

Mirrors have always retained magical significance in divination, and as lovers over the centuries stood in front of a glass preparing themselves for a love tryst they endowed the glass with all their powerful feelings about their relationship or an anticipated meeting with a new lover. It was believed that you could see the soul reflected in a mirror, not only your own but that of a future lover, even if he or she was not present. Because what you are seeing is the etheric presence of a lover, i.e. his or her spirit image called psychically in your divination, you should ideally carry out this form of divination on a Thursday, the day of Jupiter and the Norse God Thor, and one associated with shamanic out-of-body journey experiences or soul travelling (see also 'Dreaming of Love').

Traditional Mirror Marriage Divination

In medieval Europe it was believed that a single woman could see her future husband's image if she peeled an apple and combed her hair before a candle lit in front of a mirror on Hallowe'en night, one of the transition periods.

Many old spells used to reveal a true love in a mirror, not only at Hallowe'en but on any of the love festivals, involved the rhythmic, mesmeric combing of hair to lull the mind into a meditative state, especially in the moonlight. As the girl gazed into the mirror, she would softly call the lover's name, or to an unknown lover if she did not have a partner, in one of the traditional mirror chants such as:

Mirror mirror, send me
A vision pure and true,
Of he who is waiting
Over seas so blue.
Beyond the tallest mountain,

Along the village street,
Come within the glass, my love
That we therein may meet.

As the clock chimed midnight, a vision of the true love would appear in the mirror over the girl's right shoulder. This method is especially good, not just for scrying future lovers of either sex, but for any issues where you may feel uneasy or anxious about some aspect of a relationship as you may see scenes of future happiness with a partner or lover many years ahead that assure you that the love will endure.

Candle and Mirror Divination

Mirror divination can be used not only for identifying a future love, but for obtaining pictures of a relationship either now or in the future, and, more importantly since the future is not fixed, indicate potential change points that if anticipated can be used for increasing happiness. A picture of a quarrel in the mirror is not definitive, however, but indicates underlying conflicts that need to be handled sensitively, thereby changing a possible future scene for a more positive one. The most effective mirror divination method I have come across involves reflecting a horseshoe of small pink or white candles into a large oval mirror so that you cannot see the flames directly, and then shining a large pillar candle so that this is reflected in the centre of the glass.

✦ Sit to the side of the glass so that you cannot see your own reflection and leave a window open or use a small fan so that the candlelight flickers on the glass. If you want to bring the spell up to date, shine a moving fibre optic lamp into the mirror instead of the pillar candle.

◆ Position yourself so that you are looking at the candle or lamp reflected in the glass and not the candle/lamp itself.

◆ Ask a question about your love life that comes to you spontaneously, close your eyes, open them and look at the top left-hand corner of the mirror. This area represents what is moving out of your life. You may see an image, perhaps a whole scene in your mind or projected on to the glass, or hear a series of words. Each of these is a valid form of mirror scrying or gazing. Even if they are reflected in the glass, the images will only be fleeting, so do not attempt to analyse them or you will have missed the impression. Do not worry that you are imagining pictures. The imagination is the gateway between the conscious and unconscious worlds, the vehicle of the psyche, and it is where divinatory experience begins. Trust your imagination and it will take you ever further into the realms of magic and mystery.

◆ Close your eyes again, open them and look to the centre of the glass; see what is surrounding you, aspects of which may have been hidden from your conscious sight.

◆ Close your eyes for the third time, open them and look to the bottom right of the mirror at what is moving into your life. Although generally love divination reflects only the immediate future, you may see yourself with a child or yourself and your partner looking slightly older. This is only a potential future, and if your love is not there it does not mean that you have split up, merely that another aspect of your life may be to the fore.

◆ Blow out the main candle and send light to your lover.

◆ You can now write or draw the images you saw and you will find that the symbols are those that you have known from a child and that for you have a unique meaning;

make them into a story and they will answer the questions about your relationship.

Scrying in Water

This involves asking three questions about love while gazing into a rippling pool. Go to any sacred pool and you will find a tree close by. The earliest myths of many lands tell of a World Tree, the axis supporting the different worlds of existence, the heavens, the earth and the underworld, aligned by the North or Pole Star; at the foot or beneath the roots of the World Tree were two wells or pools in which you could gaze to gain knowledge of your future path.

In Viking mythology, Yggdrassil was the World Tree, an ash that supported nine worlds. Beneath the Tree were the two wells, the Well of Mimir or Knowledge for which the Father God Odin traded one of his eyes to drink of the wisdom, and the Well of the Wyrd, guarded by the three Norns or Fates who scryed in the water to determine what would occur, given the complex interaction of past, present and future which was daily being made and altered.

✦ When the Moon is full, or almost so, and shining brightly, visit a pool or lake at night that is overhung with trees: willow for the Moon Goddess, hazel for wisdom, ash for strength and healing, rowan for protection, or oak for wisdom. Identify the symbolic World Tree which may be slightly apart from the others, taller and upright, but will still be reflected in the water.

✦ If it is a clear night, find the Pole Star which marks the axis of the archetypal World Tree or use a sky globe or computer image to identify this and look up at it through the branches of your symbolic World Tree. Look down into the water, following the axis of the Pole Star, or if you cannot see it any other star directly overhead or the Moon itself. The purest visions are said to be seen in this direct line downwards, as tree and moonlight cast constantly changing patterns.

✦ Lit by the Full Moon, lakes were called Diana's mirrors, and provide a timeless tool for scrying for love. If it is a dark night you may need to supplement the natural light with tall garden candles.

✦ Find three pure white stones from as close to the pool as possible.

✦ You can ask three questions, one from each of the Fates: the first about the past and how it affects your relationship, the second about the present course of events and the third about the future. Think carefully for the questions are precious and as you formulate them you may come to understand something of your true concerns.

✦ Cast a stone into the pool, asking your question out loud, and watch the patterns of rippling light form to gain the answer. In the same way, ask questions two and three.

✦ Your questions may not be answered directly. The ancients were fond of riddles and answering one question with another, so you may receive a series of images, jumbled words, even snatches of verse or song. If these do not instantly make sense, sit quietly in the moonlight or candlelight, watching the water and not forcing any connections. They will follow naturally in dreams and over the coming days.

✦ If you do not have safe access to a pool at night, surround a large silver or clear glass bowl with pure white candles and extend over the water the branch of a willow or a similar water tree so that it casts patterns on the water.

◆ Drop three moonstones or tiny crystal quartz into the water as you voice your questions and let the images form in your mind.

— EIGHT —

Ending Love

When love ends, the sorrow is like a bereavement, with all the associated emotions of anger, regret, guilt and loss. Love poetry through the ages has expressed the agonies of infidelity, betrayal and parting in poignant words:

> *April is my mistress's face*
> *And July in her heart hath place*
> *Within her bosom is September*
> *But in her heart a cold December.*

> ANONYMOUS ITALIAN POET

The romantic poet Shelley wrote of love lost in 'The Flight of Love':

> *Its passions will rock thee,*
> *As the storms rock the ravens on high*
> *Bright reason will mock thee*
> *Like the sun from a wintry sky.*
> *From thy nest every rafter*
> *Will rot, and thine eagle home*
> *Leave thee naked to laughter*
> *When leaves fall and cold winds come.*

Whether you choose to walk away because a relationship is so destructive that you know you must go or be engulfed, whether the parting is mutual, or if you are suddenly left, betrayed, rejected and abandoned, it is almost impossible to avoid a sense of failure. Worst of all, if the ex-lover or partner is racked with guilt, perhaps for taking everything from you or abandoning you with children, he or she can do a perfect character assassination, convincing you that you deserve to be abandoned and that no one could ever find you anything other than repulsive, boring and totally inadequate. An ex-lover left me so lacking in self-confidence that, ironically, I became all the things he claimed to despise in me and it took me more than two years to re-establish any sense of self-worth. But the Sun does shine again and, like any grief, time heals, albeit slowly and not completely.

Magic can be used, not to gain revenge, for by karmic law I have seen time and time again that cruel words and vicious deeds do rebound on the sender. But ritual can banish negative feelings and doubts that freeze a betrayed lover into inaction and indecision, replaying sorrow in a never-ending cycle. These feelings can be expressed symbolically and then ritually removed, and though the spells may need to be repeated many times, each time the spell-caster becomes stronger and the pain lessens.

Even more difficult is when you are still in an abusive or emotionally draining relationship, or with a cruel or faithless lover who returns promising to be different but who reverts to destructive behaviour within weeks or even days. If you are with a controlling partner or if an ex-partner still manipulates you, perhaps through children or by interfering in your new life, you may fear that you will never be free.

Again, rituals can weaken these bonds, and you can repeat them before a potential confrontation or meeting so that you are sufficiently strong to resist emotional blackmail. Also in this chapter are details of separation ceremonies, where there are still friendly feelings or you need to see your ex and maintain a cordial relationship, either because of children or because you have to meet socially or in the work environment.

Washing Away Sorrow and Anger

Water, especially at sacred wells, has since time immemorial been used to wash away sickness and sorrow. At the Roman baths in Bath in the UK, dedicated to the Celtic-Romano goddess Sulis Minerva, lead tablets were cast into the water, expressing anger about unjust treatment, stolen property and unfair accusations. Sadly, as the lead began to dissolve, not only was the perpetrator supposedly punished but it polluted the water. The principle is valid, however, and since you may want a rather more rapid and environmentally friendly release from your negative feelings, a modern version of the ritual uses soap. It is a spell that you can use whenever pain, regret and anger engulf you.

◆ Take a miniature tablet of soap – a cheap brand of white or cream soap is fine, but you may prefer to use a cleansing soap based on eucalyptus, rosemary or tea tree which are natural purifiers.

◆ Think of a word or a visual symbol that will encapsulate your sorrow or situation. This should not be the name of your ex, because you cannot get rid of him or her without affecting your own karma; you can, however, work on freeing yourself of his or her influence.

◆ If you have a paper knife, carve the word or image on the soap; the athame or ritual knife in magic is the tool of the

Air element, giving you logic and the power of steel to cut through indecision and doubt. I have a silver knife that is shaped like a miniature sword, another tool of the Air element used in ceremonial magic. A nail file, nail, awl or any sharp metal implement will carry the same powers.

✦ When you have carved the word or symbol draw a square around it to mark the limits of the emotions and negative effects on your life to this small area.

✦ Next, etch a diagonal cross through the square and symbol. This represents the old astrological sign for Mother Earth who will absorb your pain. The act of crossing out the word or image also symbolises the removal of the angst.

✦ Fill a large bowl or bucket with very hot water and leave the soap to melt.

✦ While it is melting, do something that will give you pleasure, on the principle of replacing negative with positive, rather than leaving a void for doubts to creep back.

✦ When the soap has gone, tip the suds down a drain, saying the age-old words of those who let misery flow away in water:

Grief and sorrow, flow from me,
To the rivers, to the sea
Never more to burden me.

Repeat the ritual whenever the pain becomes intense. Deep feelings that once were love are not easily banished. Each time use an even smaller bar of soap, a good way of using up those odd slivers, and in time you will experience joy once more. This method can also be used for lessening an abusive love tie.

A Techno-Spell for Breaking Free From a Destructive or Redundant Relationship

The following spell will help you to restore a separate identity after a broken relationship, or to break away from the interference of an ex-lover. Though love spells are most usually thought of in terms of candles, herbs and flowers, and indeed many of the rituals in this book use these timeless materials, the ancient tools of magic were those most readily available to ordinary people when the spells were first cast. So in the modern world, computers can be a good tool for love magic. The magic circle drawn on the screen is no less potent than one created in the earth by a sword or wand by high magicians of old. You do not need to be a computer graphics expert to carry out this spell; the simplest images will suffice. All you will need is one of the simplest paintbox programs such as MSPaint for PCs or MacPaint for Macintoshes. Best of all is the Psion 5 pocket organiser with its user-friendly sketch tool.

✦ Work at dusk during the waning half of the Moon cycle, a good time for banishing rites.

✦ Draw two figures on the screen, not entwined but standing side by side. These can be as detailed as you wish, or just outlines.

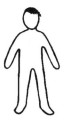 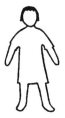

✦ Around the figures create a circle, beginning in the north of the screen and continuing in an unbroken sweep.

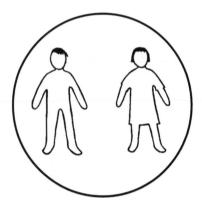

✦ Bisect the circle so that the two figures are separated by a wall. It does not matter how thin the line, but be careful you do not draw over either outline.

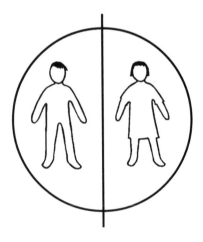

◆ Next, create two separate circles, your own first and then one around your ex-lover, again in two unbroken sweeps, saying as you create each one: *Two joined as one, now two again, separate, complete, entire, alone.*

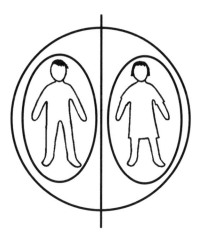

◆ Grab each circle in turn on the screen and move them further apart. Thicken the line around each circle, saying:

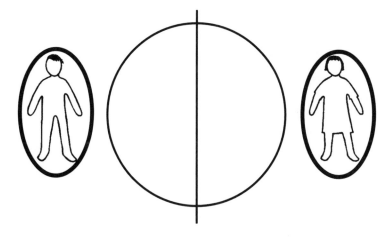

No more to touch, our spheres do move apart,
not to impinge, intrude, invade the circle now inviolate.

✦ Continue to move your lover's circle until it has disappeared from the screen, saying:

Go in peace, look no more to me,
nor think of me except as an absent friend who will not
return.

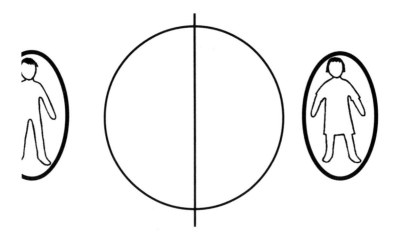

✦ Move your circle so that it is in the centre of the screen and bring it into sharp focus.

✦ Thicken the line around your circle nine times, saying:

Lingering regrets, attachments to what might have been,
do not enter my circle of self, my aura of serenity,
to hurt me with thorn and barbs, be gone.

✦ If your ex-lover is abusive or unpleasant, create a jagged edge around your circle, not to harm but merely to repel, saying:

I am myself again, complete within myself, strong and free,
having severed the links that bound me against my will.
Do not come near, you once so dear, now a memory.

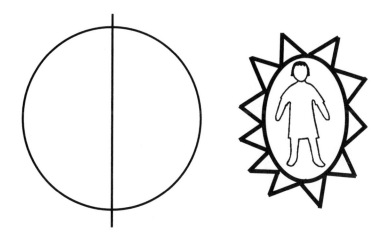

◆ You may need to repeat the ritual, which can also be used as a way of distancing yourself emotionally in an abusive relationship if circumstances demand that you cannot physically move away immediately.

(

HANDPARTING

Wiccans who separate after being joined in a handfasting ceremony sometimes have a handparting ceremony, in which they ceremonially untie the bonds that were looped between their hands, and return rings which are ritually cleansed.

But outside this tradition, and sometimes within it, the partner may have left or does not wish to enter into a reverse marriage ceremony and so it is one you can carry out alone.

In a Middle Eastern custom, a person who wishes to divorce turns three times anti-clockwise, saying: *I divorce thee, I divorce thee, I divorce thee.* This is a powerful invocation if carried out at midnight on the dark of the Moon, on the last days of the waning cycle.

The following cord ritual is much gentler, and brings healing rather than trying to apportion blame, no matter how justifiable. If you can carry it out, even if you have been badly treated, it is very liberating on a personal level. Untying cords, even if they were not used in your original marriage/joining rite, is a very potent method of externalising and marking the end of a relationship, especially if there is to be no contact between the parties concerned.

Use a diary or the weather section of a newspaper to identify the day before the New Moon. Find a tree in the garden, a healing ash, a wise hazel or a magical oak. If you do not have a garden and it is not safe to venture out into the countryside alone, use a tall wooden stool, a bedpost, banister rail at the foot of the stairs, or even a strong door handle to secure the cord.

✦ Take a long, dark red cord about nine feet (three metres) long.

✦ You can adapt curtain cord and wind it around a tree or indoor focus nine times, securing it with a very loose knot and looping the other end over your hands. Say:

We once were joined in love, we would not deny the joy we shared.
Now love grows cold and so without blame,
with only regret and sorrow for what might have been, I let you go.

✦ Unwind the cord from the tree, moving in circles further and further from the tether, chanting:

Handpart,
Dear heart,
Handfast,
Not last,
Let go,
Peace know.

✦ With a final tug, pull the knot free and then unloop your hand, saying:

Unwind,
Knot bind
No more.

✦ Light a bonfire, sprinkle cedar and rosemary herbs on it and cast the cord upon it, chanting:

Old sorrows burn,
Do not return.

✦ If you cannot light a fire, throw the cord into an incinerator or cut it into small pieces and bury it, saying:

Sorrows decay,
come no more my way.

✦ To end the ceremony, turn three times anti-clockwise, saying:

I unbind thee,
I unwind thee,
Joy find thee.

✦ If you are working with your ex-partner, use separate cords knotted together around the tree.

A Healing Ritual

This ritual aims to let the bad parts of a relationship decay, while preserving happy memories. If you were together for many years, especially if the parting was against your will, there is so much shared life and memory. You do not wish to banish what may have been happy years for they are a part of you, and they, along with your present sorrow, have made you the person you are now: wiser, perhaps more compassionate, and able to use that experience to create an even more fulfilling future. Our ancestors who hung rags on trees around healing wells and let them decay, having dipped the rag in the well and bound it round the affliction, understood that miracle cures were rare and that time was of the essence; also that it was necessary to detach the pain so that the system might be restored to health.

Today, you can still see rags and ribbons around wells, and you can take a dark-coloured ribbon representing pain to a healing well, dip it in the water and hang it on a tree, making sure the ribbon is biodegradable. Alternatively, you can name a dying flower for the pain and bury it close to the well or in your garden.

The following ritual evolved while I was working on a BBC TV programme with a man who had literally been stabbed through the heart, leaving him with a vast aftermath of unresolved emotion. We cannot go back to what we were before a painful experience, but we can bury the pain and, taking what is positive even from the most traumatic experiences, create new growth and life.

'Burying the bone' to represent a quarrel, like burying meat to represent an illness, is one of the oldest forms of magic and works on the principle of decay, which then becomes the source of new life in the soil.

◆ Take a plum, peach, pear or apple and wash it in water that has been left in a mesh-covered crystal or glass container for a full Sun and Moon cycle. Water from a sacred spring is a good basis for magical water. Before using it, sprinkle five grains of salt into the water.

◆ Place the fruit in a flower bed in the early morning as the sun is rising, saying: *As this fruit decays, so will my sorrow and anger grow less until they are no more.*

◆ Wait for the stone to take root, but as this is such a slow process, plant a fragrant fast-growing herb garden to surround your buried fruit: rosemary for remembrance of earlier joys, lavender for reconciliation and peace, mint for cleansing and new energies, sage for wisdom, chamomile for quiet sleep and healing, and lemon balm for new love (see also 'The Plants of Love').

◆ Whenever you doubt, inhale the wonderful fragrance of your new hopes, and one day a tiny shoot of your tree may come through the earth – or you may have moved on and your life be bearing fruit of its own.

◆ If you do not have a garden, you can plant your fruit in a large pot or window box and transplant the seedling later.

(

A FORMAL DIVORCE OR SEPARATION CEREMONY

In the modern world formal rites of passage, apart from wedding ceremonies and funerals, are largely missing from our lives, especially if we do not belong to one of the traditional faiths. Yet rites of passage were ways of openly acknowledging the transition from one stage of life to another, and the actions undertaken and the words spoken externalised previously unexpressed yet keenly felt emotions. It is when these remain unacknowledged that depression or the desire for revenge can surface.

Until the 1950s divorce was relatively uncommon, because it was difficult legally and regarded as a social stigma, and this resulted in heartbreak for those locked in loveless unions. Now that one in three marriages ends this way, as well as the numerous statistically unrecorded relationships in which the couple are married in all but name, few of us will avoid the ending of at least one significant relationship.

Clergy will now perform divorce ceremonies, sometimes attended by those who witnessed the original marriage, but with the vast increase in secular rather than religious weddings, such ceremonies will more usually be personally initiated without any official participation. Such a ritual can be especially helpful on the actual day of divorce or official parting, which however amicable is like a death; the loss of all the future years together that now will never be. Rituals are in us all and if we follow our hearts and instincts we know what to do and what to say.

✦ Prepare a place with flowers, if possible of the kind used at the original betrothal, on a table containing any symbols of the love: jewellery given, rings, even love letters tied together with ribbon, plus any special photographs that were of significance. You will need salt, incense of myrrh or sandalwood for healing emotional wounds, and scented water.

✦ Place the symbols of the former relationship in the centre of the table, surrounded by a circle of flowers, with a small pottery dish of salt to the north of the table outside the circle.

✦ Set the incense to the east and a small glass dish of water to the west, again outside the circle.

✦ Stand in front of the table, facing north.

✦ Outside the circle, to the south, place a large white, cream or pale yellow pillar candle. Beeswax will release a gentle healing aroma as it burns. This candle represents the union of the couple.

✦ Light this candle either singly or with your partner, using two tapers joined in the candle wick, saying:

Because we were joined in love/marriage,
I/we light this uniting candle as a token of what we shared,
joining ourselves for the last time in this light.

✦ Using the same tapers, light two smaller white candles from the central candle. Place one on either side of the large one. If you are working alone, first light the left-hand candle for yourself and then light the second by proxy. Say:

The light divides but is not diminished.
I am what I am and you are what you are.
Not us, you are yourself once more and I am myself as the old light dims and dies.

✦ The first candle is extinguished by one or both simultaneously and a silent wish made for the other's happiness.

✦ If children are present, it can be reassuring if you and the divorcing partner can light a pure white parental candle from your separate candles. This candle can replace the original unity candle and should be lit with the same tapers, saying:

*We kindle this lesser flame of unity in affection and friend-
ship for we will always be united in the love of the children
we created and nurtured together,
we pledge ourselves to put aside any personal differences as
we continue to care for them jointly, so willingly and with
continuing pride and wonder of what we did achieve in their
creation.*

◆ The children may want to add lighted tapers momentarily
to the family flame, and this can be rekindled at family
occasions when the divorced couple come together.
Alternatively, you can use a multi-wicked candle for the
family unity flame, so that each child lights one of the
wicks, the first and second being lit by the parent/s.

◆ Take the salt and sprinkle a few grains over the love
symbols, waft the incense six times clockwise, and finally
sprinkle scented water, saying:

*I consecrate these symbols of former love with the powers of
Earth, Air, Fire and Water,
purifying them of all anger and bad intent, so that they can
remain signs of what was once so pure and true.*

◆ If you are working alone, place the symbols wrapped in
silk in a wooden box to form a memory box; if you are
both present, pre-arrange what each would like to keep of
these sentimental tokens. Avoid any dispute souring the
occasion.

◆ Present your partner with a small wooden box engraved
with his/her name containing the former love tokens.
You may decide to send an ex-partner an item you know
he/she values on a sentimental level as a gesture of peace,
even if he or she is absent.

✦ If there is bitterness, as you separate the marriage flame into two, ask the benign powers of the universe that your former partner's heart may be softened, and that if there are children that you may still be as one in your love of them. Catch some of the melting wax and make a heart, and as it begins to set, rejoin it to the candle.

The Festivals of Love and Fertility

In times when most people lived in the countryside, the natural world formed the arena for love and fertility festivals that marked the passing year and mirrored the corresponding rise and fall of natural energies that flow through humans as well as animals. These festivals were once dedicated to the old solar and nature deities and to the Earth Mother; with the advent of Christianity the names of these were changed to those of saints and Archangels, but in essence the festivals continued as a focus for the fertility of land and people and the love matches that were made under their auspices, as they had for hundreds or even thousands of years. For example, St John's Eve and day on June 23 and 24 absorbed the slightly earlier Summer Solstice rites, while St Michael, Archangel of the Sun, whose day is close to the Autumn Equinox, presided over Harvest Home rituals.

In earlier times, the fertility of the people and the fertility of the soil were inextricably linked. Couples made love in the woods or fields at times of sowing or peak growth times, re-enacting the Sacred Marriage between the Sky Father or Horned God and Earth Mother, symbolically fertilising the crops as well as ensuring their own fecundity. In the Mid-West of the US, a token plant set by a pregnant woman was and still is believed to ensure the success of the whole crop, while in Indonesia rice crops are traditionally encouraged to produce the maximum amount of seed by a couple making love in the fields at the time the rice is blooming.

Scientific research gives this apparently two-way fertility connection some credence. In 'Love Divination', I suggested that we could unconsciously influence the growth of plants to guide us to a decision. Pierre Savon from New Jersey, USA, investigated extra-sensory perception in plants. He discovered that there would be an electronic reaction on a tone oscillator attached to his plants at the same time as he was making love with his girlfriend eighty miles away. The moment of orgasm produced the most dramatic response.

Further research explains how the merriment and unbridled lovemaking of the old festivals were conducive to conception. A team from the University of Cardiff, led by Jacky Boivin of the School of Biology, found that women retained more active sperm when sex had been pleasurable. The difference may be crucial for some couples who are having difficulty conceiving because of low fertility. In such couples lovemaking frequently occurs under stressful conditions as it is determined by the clinical fertile period rather than sexual desire. Researchers found that women who rated sex highly, including having an orgasm, retained more sperm in the cervix. There were two main theories to explain the possible link. The team suggested that the spasms in orgasm may draw in the sperm, while Dr Boivin was quoted as saying that: 'Arousal has been shown to reduce the acidic environment of the vagina. This is important as the pH balance in the cervix has been shown to impact on the sperm's survival.'

With the coming of the Industrial Revolution, many people moved from the countryside and worked by the clock rather than the sun; holidays were no longer governed by the agricultural year, but confined to a single week in the height of summer when machinery was being serviced. The advent of artificial light meant that darkness no longer heralded rest, lovemaking and sleep, while the heat of the factories and the mills took away an awareness of temperature changes, where formerly people would toil less when the earth was frozen and so regain their energies for the long hours of tilling in summer and for the harvest. The flowers and herbs that grew in the hedgerows were no longer so accessible and with the widespread increase of literacy in later Victorian times, the family oral herb and flower lore, and their magical love and fertility as well as healing associations, were replaced by more formal channels for medical and emotional problems. Many indigenous people, including the Native Americans, believe that when the sacred circle or hoop is broken, humankind becomes alienated from their surroundings and ultimately from themself, and so artificial stimulants and medical intervention sometimes become necessary to restore libido.

However, it is still possible to harness the rising energies of spring and summer to attract love and fertility; rituals practised on the ebbing year are no less valuable in reaffirming established partnerships, bringing love in mature years, or effecting a reconciliation in a relationship after a period of coldness or estrangement. These ebbing energies counter the increasing tendency to give up rather than work through problems in a relationship or to overreact to difficulties.

For the purpose of this chapter, I have divided the energy patterns into the four conventional seasons, spring, summer, autumn and winter, each of which incorporates two of the Celtic eightfold year divisions shared by the northern magical tradition that extended through Scandinavia and northern and eastern Europe as far as Russia; the Mediterranean regions celebrate similar festivals. People now living in Australia, America or South Africa, whose ancestors came from these colder regions, may still feel the call of spring at the time their forebears would have been celebrating the Spring Equinox.

Some of the rituals are interchangeable, especially those which occur as part of the three central spring and summer fertility/love rituals. So, although eggs are associated with Easter and the Spring Equinox, they are central to all fertility rituals as a symbol of incubating new life. Mix and match the spells and take what is of use to create your own rituals.

Spring Energies for New Love and Increasing Commitment

Early Spring Energies

Early spring energies last from January 30 until around March 21, the Spring Equinox, which varies slightly according to the calendar. These powers are good for attracting love, for nurturing a new love, for learning to trust a new lover after a failed relationship, for romance and for first love. You can adapt these rituals at any time of the year or to your own region's calendar for spells for new love and trust.

For our forebears, because infant mortality and death in childbirth were so high, the urgency to reproduce began at the first spring festival and lasted through to late summer, and so even the first spring had its earthier elements. But the energies of this period truly belong to St Valentine, whose benevolence can perhaps rekindle the art of gentle love and chaste courtship that give couples a chance to know and trust each other without the pressure of consummating their relationship in the early days.

Brigantia, Imbolc or Oimelc

This Celtic festival of Ewe's Milk was held from sunset on January 31 until sunset on February 2. It was the first festival of the Celtic spring when the early lambs were born and so fresh milk was available after the long winter. The original Brigit, Brighde or Brigid, is celebrated at this festival; the maiden aspect of the Triple Goddess.

On Bride's Eve, January 31, a bride's bed of straw, decorated with ribbons and the first spring flowers, was made in front of the fire in the main farm or house of an area and the inhabitants would shout: 'Bride, come in, your bed is ready.' The symbolic bride maiden would leave her cows and a cauldron at the door, bringing in peace and plenty. Originally, as I described earlier, this was the time of the deflowering of the maiden goddess by the chief of the tribe.

Milk and honey were poured over the bride bed by the women of the household. The menfolk were summoned and, having paid either a coin, a flower posy, or a kiss, would enter the circle of firelight and ask for help with their craft or agriculture and make a wish on the bride bed.

February 14, St Valentine's Day

This is perhaps the best-known festival of lovers, and falling close to Brigantia reflects the romantic, courtly, idealised aspect of young and new love that developed in the Middle Ages.

St Valentine was, according to legend, a young priest who defied an edict of the Emperor Claudius II that soldiers should not be allowed to marry as it made them poor fighters. St Valentine conducted the weddings of a number of young soldiers and was executed on February 14, AD 269, thereafter becoming the patron saint of lovers. It is said that while Valentine was in prison, he restored the sight of the jailer's blind daughter and that she fell in love with him.

Legend adds that as he was taken to be executed, he wrote on the wall a message for his love: 'Always, your Valentine.'

I have read alternative versions of the story, but none which is quite so romantic.

It is also the day on which birds are said to choose their mates, according to Chaucer's *Parliament of The Fowles*:

For this was on St Valentine's Day
When every Fowl cometh to choose her mate.

If an unmarried girl saw a bird during the morning of February 14, it was believed that she would divine her future love. Most Valentine rituals were devised in less liberated days when the ambition of every maid was to find a husband.

If you see a hen and cockerel together early on St Valentine's Day, it is a sign that you will be married. The number of animals you see as you leave home will tell you how many months will elapse before the nuptials take place. The old myths also promise that if a girl sees a crow, she will marry a clergyman; a robin, a sailor; a goldfinch, a millionaire; any yellow bird, someone who is well off; a sparrow, love in a cottage; a bluebird, poverty; and a crossbill, quarrels. A wryneck portends that she will remain an old maid and a flock of doves promises happiness in every way.

One custom that has died out is that no lover should step over the threshold on Valentine's morn without wearing a yellow crocus, the flower of St Valentine, that is said to bring luck in love.

It was also believed that the first man an unattached maiden spied on Valentine's morning would be her true love. However, any maiden who wanted a glimpse of her future husband had already visited the local churchyard on Valentine's Eve, and as the clock struck twelve she would run around the church, calling:

I sow hemp seed,
Hemp seed I sow,
He that loves me,
Come after me and mow.

Brigantia crystals   Garnet, bloodstone, amethyst, rose quartz and moonstone.

Flowers, incense and herbs of Brigantia   Angelica, basil, benzion, crocus, celandine, heather, myrrh and snow-drop.

Brigantia candle colours   White, cream and pink or any pastel colour for unfolding love and tenderness.

((

AN EARLY SPRING RITUAL FOR NURTURING NEW LOVE

This is a cold weather version of the eastern European custom of planting marigolds in the soil from a lover's footprint to encourage the growth of faithful love.

◆ Find a quantity of snow; newly fallen snow, especially in the early morning light, is best of all. If necessary, you can use powdery, slightly melting ice from a freezer.

◆ If fresh snow, wait for your lover to walk in it (send him or her out to look for the cat) or secretly borrow his or her shoe to make an imprint. Now place your own footprint to almost cover but not obliterate your lover's, saying: *Let us walk a while in the other's shoes that our minds may be in harmony.*

- If you cannot obtain a footprint, imprint a serrated metal dish in the ice or snow – you can buy heart-shaped ones for making novelty cakes – and draw your entwined initials in the snow shape with a stick.

- Scoop the imprinted snow or ice into a silver-coloured pitcher and leave it in a warm place to melt naturally. Stir it nine times clockwise, saying: *Affection flow, in tenderness grow, that we may be as one eternally.*

- Take a small quantity of earth. If the snow is soft, dig some from the hole left by the footprint; otherwise take it from your garden or window box.

- Plant two daffodil or hyacinth bulbs in a pot so that they will flower in a few weeks' time, around the Spring Equinox, running your fingers through the soil as you pat it round the bulbs, saying: *Flower and bloom and with it our love.*

- When the ice has melted, water the bulbs, saying:

  Joined in snow and cold may we walk together in trust and affection in shadow as well as sunlit moments,
  sharing what we have and not regretting what we have not.

- Sprinkle a little of the snow water on the plants each day until the bulbs are grown. If they do not prosper it does not mean your love is doomed, only that it may need more nurturing. Sometimes the slowest growth leads to the surest foundations.

Late Spring Energies

Late spring energies run from around March 21 until April 30. This is a good time for making a serious commitment, for consummating a relationship, for all new phases within an existing relationship, for setting up home with another person, and perhaps for planning a family. But you can use its rituals and energies at any time of the year when you enter the late spring of a relationship.

The Spring or Vernal Equinox or Ostara Time

The Spring Equinox lasts for three days from sunset on March 21 until sunset on March 23, or thereabouts according to the calendar. The Sacred Marriage between Earth and Sky was practised in many cultures at the time of spring; in Ancient Babylon, the Sacred Marriage took place each year between the God Tammuz and the Goddess Ishtar. The festival of Akitu or Zag-Mug celebrated the rising of the waters of the Tigris, followed by the Euphrates, and the coming of the spring rains to bring fertility at the Spring Equinox. Like many of the harvest gods, he died every year and was fetched from the underworld by his consort who restored him to life. And so the energies of the Spring Equinox may help a couple conceive a child.

It is the time of year when, in the old Celtic tradition, the God of light overcame the God of darkness and marked the coming of days that were longer than night. The first eggs of spring were painted and offered on the shrine of the Anglo-Saxon Goddess Eostre or the Norse Ostara to whom the hare was sacred (this is the origin of the Easter rabbit). Easter is the Christian celebration most closely associated with the Spring Equinox; wake at dawn on Equinox morn or Easter Sunday and, it is said, you can see the Sun or, in the Christian tradition, angels dancing in a stream or river.

Spring Equinox crystals Citrine, yellow beryl, yellow calcite, yellow rutilated quartz with streaks of gold for growth to come, and all shades of fluorite.

Flowers, incense and herbs of Spring Equinox Cedar, celandine, cinquefoil, crocus, daffodil, honeysuckle, pine, primrose, sage, tansy, thyme and violet.

Spring Equinox candle colours Use yellow and green for the clear light from the east and the budding vegetation.

((

A Late Spring Equinox Ritual for Pledging Commitment

If possible, spend the night before the ritual camping with your partner in a forest or staying in a hotel near woods, so that even if you cannot make love outdoors, you are close to trees, symbol of male potency. If you are indoors, light Equinox Eve candles after dusk.

✦ During the late afternoon, pick or buy six yellow spring flowers; place them in water, stirred six times clockwise with a stick from a tree branch to awaken the energies.

✦ Wake before dawn and go with your lover to the nearest running water, symbol of female creative power. Take with you the six flowers, the number of Venus.

✦ Just as dawn breaks, each of you should cast a flower into the water at the same time, making a silent pledge to the other.

✦ Cast the third bloom into the water repeating aloud your own silent pledge.

✦ Let your lover cast the fourth flower, repeating his or her silent pledge aloud.

- For the fifth flower, take on your lover's pledge and speak it to him/her, and as the sixth bloom is cast into the water he/she can echo back your pledge to you.

- As the light finally breaks through, hold hands and look together into the water, seeing not angels or the Sun dancing, but yourselves joined and blessed by the ascending light. If you are lucky, the sun may cast a halo around you both in the water.

- Consummate your love, if possible in the open air under the trees, and spend the day making plans for the future.

- Try and make this a special anniversary and renewal of your private vows.

Summer Energies for Fertility and Male Sexual Power

Early Summer Energies

Early summer energies run from April 30 until around June 21, the Summer Solstice or Longest Day, which varies slightly according to the calendar. This period is good for sex magic, making a commitment in the eyes of the world, and because it was the time of woodland weddings, for marriage, especially a first marriage. As the middle fertility festival it is also the most potent for conceiving a child. But you can use its rituals at any time of the year or in your own region's calendar for sex, marriage or fertility.

Beltain or Beltane: the Coming of Early Summer
Beltain runs for three days from sunset on April 30 until sunset on May 2, and marks the beginning of the Celtic

summer when cattle were released from barns and driven between twin fires to cleanse them and ritually endow them with fertility. Young men and girls would leap naked over the fires before spending the night of May Eve together in the woodlands looking for the first May (hawthorn) blossoms to decorate the houses.

The maypoles, some of which were 40 feet or more high, formed the focus of love and fertility dances on May morning. Red, blue, green, yellow and white ribbons, representing the union of earth and sky, winter and summer, water and fire, were entwined and girls bathed their faces in the potent dew. The Beltain celebration was in essence a festival of sexual pleasure as nature blossomed.

Because of the connection between the fertility of the soil and human fertility, fruits, flowers and herbs were regarded as appropriate symbols of fertility. Among the Kara-Kirgiz people of Turkmenistan, barren women would roll themselves on the ground under a solitary apple tree in order to become pregnant. In northern India, coconuts are considered fertility symbols and are sacred to Sri, Goddess of prosperity. They are kept in shrines, blessed and given by priests to women who wish to conceive. Finally, the Guarani Indians of South America believe that if a woman eats a double grain of millet she will become a mother of twins.

Beltain crystals Clear crystal quartz, golden tiger's eye, amber and topaz.

Flowers, incense and herbs of Beltain Almond, angelica, ash, cowslip, frankincense, hawthorn, lilac, marigold and rose.

Beltain candle colours Silver and red, also green to reflect the blossoming of the greenery and to recall Jack O'Green, or the Green Man, the old God of vegetation who is associated with Robin Hood and who married the May Queen.

An Early Summer Ritual for Opening Yourself to the Fertility Energies

When you hope to conceive a child, whether through love-making, IVF or artificial insemination, you can tune into the natural fertility energies that run through your body as well as the earth, but which may have become blocked.

✦ At dawn on May morn, use an eye dropper to collect the first dew, if possible from an oak tree, considered in myth to be the semen of the gods.

✦ If you cannot find dew, use any flower essence associated with fertility, for example the Deva essences basil, hibiscus or martagon lily.

✦ Place your dew or flower essence in a small clear glass phial.

✦ Take a small perfect almond or walnut, symbols of the female ovum. Walnuts are still thrown at the bride in some European countries to endow her with fertility.

✦ Place the walnut and phial of dew side by side in the sunlight, or if it is a dark day, light a large orange candle between them.

✦ Next, take a perfect white oval egg and with a needle make a hole to remove the yolk and white. Use these in cooking, or if you do not eat eggs feed them to an animal so that they are not wasted. Split the shell in half. Alternatively, you can use an egg made of cardboard, wood or china that has two halves.

- Place the walnut gently in the egg and hold the needle up to the Sun or pass it through the candle flame.

- Gently pierce the walnut, place it in one half of the egg and sprinkle it with the dew or flower essence, saying:

    Sky and earth unite in love; so began the world as light moved over the waters.
    May we be allowed to play our part in continuing the sacred chain line of life.

- Bind the other half of the egg to the half containing the fertilised walnut with ribbons of red, blue, green, white and yellow, and bury it at the foot of an oak or ash, both World Trees, or under a faery tree, like hawthorn, or a piece of land at a location that is of great significance to you, perhaps where you first made love.

- Make love when you wish during the day. Afterwards, spend time weaving together the story of the child you hope to create in love, for in a sense the potential child comes into being every time you and a partner make love.

Later Summer Energies

Later summer energies run from around June 21 until July 31, Lammas or Lughnassadh. These energies are good for male potency, for marriages and permanent commitments second time around, the love of experience, and also for sex magic and sacred sexuality. As the third fertility festival, the culmination of male/female energies from the previous two festivals can be of help if you have experienced difficulty conceiving a child, if only in dissolving the barriers of anxiety caused by trying all spring and summer without success. The energies can also be harnessed when any of these situations arise at other times in the year.

Summer Solstice or Midsummer Magic

The Summer Solstice runs from sunset on the Solstice Eve, June 20 or thereabouts, for three days. The Summer Solstice marks the high point of the year, the Longest Day, and is the zenith of light and of magic. Modern Druids still celebrate this festival of light with ceremonies at midnight on Solstice Eve and at dawn and noon of the actual Solstice day. Traditionally, great fire wheels were rolled down the hillsides in honour of the triumph of the old Sun gods and were continued as part of the Midsummer festivals when the summer celebrations fell under the auspices of St John.

According to tradition, the yellow herb St John's Wort, which first blooms at Midsummer, should be picked at midnight on Midsummer Eve (June 23) by a woman wishing to become pregnant. She should walk naked alone in a garden and speak not a word. She must then sleep with the plant under her pillow and within nine months should have a child. However, there was competition for the herb. Unmarried maidens would gather St John's Wort after dusk on the same eve without eating anything all day and, it was said, they would have a husband before the year was out. If they then slept with the yellow plant under their pillow, dreams of true love were promised.

It was also the time when girls made their Midsummer Men to assure themselves of a virile lover. Clay was gathered on Midsummer Eve as dusk was falling. St John's Wort, trefoil and sprigs of rue were gathered and the shape of a man drawn in a circle on the clay; in earlier times this would have horns for the Horned God. The herbs of Midsummer were pressed into the figure and it was left facing east to catch the Solstice sunrise that would empower it. If the herbs survived, it was a promising omen of many nights of passion.

Summer Solstice crystals Amber, carnelian, jasper, lapis lazuli and turquoise for male potency.

Flowers, incense and herbs of Summer Solstice Chamomile, dill, elder, fennel, lavender, rue, St John's Wort, trefoil, vervain and verbena.

Summer Solstice candle colours Gold or orange to mirror the Sun at its height.

((

A SUMMER SOLSTICE MALE POTENCY RITUAL

For thousands of years, lodestones were placed in a love-inducing oil such as sandalwood or passion flower, and after twenty-four hours the infusion was rubbed on the penis before making love. But even well diluted in a very gentle oil such as almond, the carrier oil of fertility, direct application to the genitals does require caution. I would substitute lavender or rose, which are very gentle and mild, using no more than five drops to 30ml of almond essential or flower oil. However, using contagious magic you can transfer the potency from the charged lodestone without direct body contact with the oil.

✦ At dawn on the Solstice, take a pointed lodestone and place it downwards in a round ceramic bowl.

✦ Sprinkle a potency oil such as sandalwood or ylang-ylang, mixed with three parts of almond, over the lodestone. Alternatively, ask your partner to do this.

✦ Rub the oil vertically from the bottom to the top of the inverted lodestone, visualising successful lovemaking.

- Leave the lodestone still in the bowl in the light until noon when you should place it in a red drawstring bag with a turquoise or dyed blue howzite crystal (both male power stones) and keep it beneath the mattress while making love at noon on the Solstice. You can carry out this ritual at other times of the year, but always begin at dawn.

Autumn Energies for Reconciliation

Early Autumn Energies

Early autumn energies run from July 31 until around September 22, and are good for uniting against outside inter-ference or pressures, for settling disputes within a relationship, especially over family members, and for middle-aged marriages and love affairs.

Lammas or Lughnassadh: the First Corn and Wheat Harvest

Lammas runs from sunset on July 31 until sunset on August 2. This is the Feast of Lugh, Celtic God of light, and grandson of the Sun, the first harvest festival to give thanks to the earth for her bounty.

It was considered unlucky to cut down the last sheaf of corn as this was thought to represent the Corn God who was willingly offering his life in sacrifice that the cycle of life, death and rebirth, planting, growth and harvesting might continue. Harvesters would simultaneously hurl their sickles at the last sheaf so no one knew who had killed the Corn God. This last sheaf was then made into a corn dolly, symbol of the Earth Mother, and decorated with the scarlet ribbons of Cerridwen, the Celtic Mother Goddess. It would be hung over the hearth throughout winter.

As Lammas was a time for feasting and meeting for distant members of the tribe, it was the perfect occasion for marriages and for all matters of justice and resolving disputes, as the roads were sufficiently dry for circuit judges, originally the Druids, to visit remote settlements.

Trial marriages were frequently set up at Lammas. The young couple would thrust their hands through a holed stone and agree to stay together for a year and a day. The following Lammas they could renew the arrangement or stand back to back and walk away from one another, bringing the 'marriage' to a formal close. Some Wiccan practitioners still dedicate their marriages for a year and a day, which does not represent a lack of commitment, but the opportunity to annually renew vows by choice, rather than legal statute.

Lammas or Lughnassadh crystals Tiger's eye, fossilised woods, rutilated quartz, agates of all kinds, especially banded.

Flowers, incense and herbs of Lammas Cedarwood, cinnamon, fenugreek, ginger and heather, myrtle and sunflower.

Lammas candle colours Dark orange and yellow to reflect the coming of autumn.

((

A LAMMAS RITUAL

This is good for settling a long-running emotional dispute within a relationship. Every marriage has its potentially explosive areas that can break out during even a minor disagreement, whether over teenage children, in-laws, ex-partners or lovers, colleagues at work or friends. The practical aspects, money and property, fall under the auspices of the late winter period.

The ancients would bury the bone, quite literally etching a symbol on a bone and placing it in Mother Earth to absorb and rework as new life.

First you need to lay the issue to rest. In 'Fidelity and Lasting Love', I mentioned a candle ritual for clearing the air. This time you are going to reverse roles and take each other's part, as though acting as advocate in a Lammas justice court.

✦ Mark the top half of a small dark orange beeswax Lammas candle with two notches about 3cm each. Burn cedarwood incense or oil for calm and light the candle, extinguishing any other light.

✦ Surround the candle with ears of corn or dried grasses and place it on a fireproof tray. Light the candle together, using two tapers that join in the flame.

✦ Let your partner talk uninterrupted about your difficulties and point of view while you try to see where the argument is flawed.

✦ When the candle is burned through the first section, he or she should make a corn or grass knot and burn it in the flame, repeating the age-old banishing chant: *Tangle the anger, tangle the pain, by this flame make me free again.*

✦ Next, you should speak as advocate, seeing the situation through your partner's eyes, and when your time is through, likewise tangle and burn your anger in the candle flame, repeating the chant.

✦ Sit by candlelight recalling all the happy times in your relationship, but do not refer to the 'bone' of contention.

✦ When the candle is burned through, draw a square in the wax, mark a cross through it and bury it either in the garden or near a field of barley, corn or wheat. As it is pure beeswax it will not harm the environment. You may need to repeat the ritual regularly.

Later Autumn Energies

Later autumn energies run from around 22 September until 31 October and are good for reconciliation after a bad quarrel or a separation, and for healing the emotional wounds caused by betrayal or coldness.

The Autumn Equinox

The Autumn Equinox or Time of Gathering runs for three days from sunset on 22 September or thereabouts. It was traditionally celebrated as the second 'wild or green harvest', a time of celebration for the fruits and vegetables of the earth and any remaining crops, originally dedicated to the Earth Mother. On the day when equal night and day heralded winter, the feast formed a sympathetic magical gesture to ensure that there would be enough food during the winter, through the display and consumption of the finest of the harvest. It is also a time when the Sky and Animal God is said to retreat for the long winter. Druids climb to the top of a hill to take leave of the summer Sun as the nights will get longer.

And so it is a time for looking backwards to what has been, and forwards to what will be, accepting what was lost or spoiled in the harvest and rejoicing in what has survived.

Autumn Equinox crystals Blue lace agate, blue beryl or azurite, moss agate, jade.

Flowers, incense and herbs of Autumn Equinox Ferns, geranium, myrrh, pine and Solomon's Seal.

Autumn Equinox candle colours Blue for the autumn rain and green for the Earth Mother and the wild harvest.

An Equinox Ritual for Forgiveness

This can also be used to acknowledge or accept frailty in others.

✦ Pile a bowl high with autumn berries, nuts or seeds and surround it with autumn leaves on small branches.

✦ Burn eucalyptus or tea tree oil for cleansing and geranium for the increase of love.

✦ Light a blue candle for the purifying rain and green for the nurturing mother who transforms what is redundant into new life.

✦ Sit either alone or, if possible, with your lover and say:

What is lost and what is gained balance out,
the riches of the harvest and the dying of the leaves as day
and night are equal.

✦ Pick an autumn leaf, saying: *As leaves die, so will new ones in the ripe time grow. So is it with love.*

✦ Let your partner pick a berry, nut or seed and eat it, saying: *As fruit ripens, it brings joy and takes away bitterness. So is it with love.*

✦ He/she then takes a leaf and you a berry, repeating the appropriate words. Continue to pluck leaves and eat berries alternately until all are gone.

✦ Make a pile of the leaves as you work in a rush or wicker basket and when the ritual is finished extinguish the candles and oil.

✦ Go together to a high place and let the leaves fly free in the wind, saying:

Fly away sorrow, fly away anger,
what is lost and what is gained fly free, to be reborn in the
spring.

✦ Run down the hill as fast as you can, feeling yourselves free to love again.

✦ You can carry out this ritual at other times of the year, using paper flowers or leaves if there are no autumn ones, or alone to pave the way for a reconciliation.

Winter Energies

These are best used for family matters and for presevering in darker times.

Early Winter Energies

Early winter energies run from 31 October until around 21 December, the Winter Solstice or Shortest Day (which varies slightly according to the calendar). These times are good for family matters, whether the family is a couple, a couple with children, a single parent, a family with step and adoptive members or an extended family of several generations, for older love matches and for keeping a mature relationship loving and joyous. Again, you can use these rituals at any time of the year or in your own region's calendar when family concerns fill your heart.

Samhain or Hallowe'en

Samhain, which runs roughly from sunset on 31 October to sunset on 2 November means 'summer's end'. Hallowe'en, or the Eve of All Hallows in the Christian calendar, has become a night of ghouls, ghosts and plastic skeletons. This festival marked the beginning of the Celtic New Year and a time when family members who had been tending the cattle on the hills would return and be welcomed home for the winter. The Celts also believed that the family dead could be welcomed back for this special night. And it was a time for looking into the future, especially for matters of love.

Although Hallowe'en no longer marks the transition between one year and the next, the barriers between past, present and future are still regarded as especially close on this night and so it is an auspicious time for divination, especially concerning love which was its chief focus until comparatively recently.

Much of the written evidence for Hallowe'en love divination comes from a poem, 'Hallowe'en', by Scotland's great bard Robert Burns. In this we learn that if a young man eats a raw or roasted salted herring before bedtime, in his dreams his future wife will bring a drink to quench the thirst of the dreamer. Burns also reveals that a blindfolded young girl is led out to the cabbage patch to pull up a cabbage. The amount of dirt clinging to the roots indicates the size of the dowry; the shape and size of the cabbage foretells the appearance and height of her intended. She must then nibble the raw heart and its flavour and sweetness will reveal her future husband's disposition. She then takes the stalk home and puts it behind the outer door. The first person to call in the morning will be her future husband.

In another traditional Hallowe'en ritual, a maiden should go to a kiln and throw a bobbin of blue yarn in the pot, all the time winding it on to a new bobbin. Suddenly she will feel someone hold the thread and if she calls: 'Who holds my yarn?', her future love will answer his name.

Samhain crystals Sodalite, dark amethyst, smoky quartz, deep brown jasper and jet and obsidian (apache tear). Hold your apache tear up to the candle and see the light shine through promising that any sorrows or setbacks will not last for ever.

Flowers, incense and herbs of Samhain Cypress, dittany, ferns, nutmeg, sage, and pine.

Samhain candle colours Black, navy blue or deep purple for letting go of fear, and orange for the joy of immortality that is promised at this time.

☾

A Samhain Ritual for Keeping Loved Ones Safe

If you have a hearth in your home, set the ritual there, but you can create one for the purpose of the ritual using a circle of bricks set against a wall indoors or out.

✦ Gather you lover and any family members who will not feel uneasy and let them sit or kneel in a circle around the hearth.

✦ Place a dish of salt for the protection of the earth at the back of the hearth to represent symbolic north, a circle of cypress or sage incense sticks for the protection of the air to the right, a deep purple candle for the protection of fire to the south of the hearth, and a dish of water in which a smoky quartz has been soaked for twelve hours for protective energies to the left. You can leave the crystal in the water if you wish. You have now created an elemental circle of protection.

✦ Take the salt and scatter a circle clockwise, beginning at the back of the hearth, around the circle of your loved ones, saying:

Within the circle of protection, let none harm you, by thought, word or deed, by the power of this salt, gift of Mother Earth who casts her mantle over all.

✦ Return the salt to the hearth and taking one of the incense sticks in a container, make a clockwise circle of smoke around your loved ones, beginning at the back of the hearth, saying:

Within this circle of protection, let none harm you by thought, word or deed, by the power of this incense, gift of Father Sky whose thunderbolts and mighty winds drive away all that may do hurt.

✦ Return the incense to the hearth, take the candle and beginning once more at the back, make a circle clockwise in the air around your loved ones, saying:

Within this circle of protection, let none harm you by thought, word or deed, by the power of this fire, gift of Brother Sun who shines light and warmth upon this circle of love.

✦ Return the candle to the hearth and finally take up the water, sprinkling a circle around the family, saying:

Within this circle of protection, let none harm you by thought, word or deed, by the power of Sister Water who encloses you on a magical island of security.

✦ Return the water to the hearth and touch each of the elements in turn, saying:

Earth, Air, Fire, Water, cast your circle wherever my loved ones are, be it across oceans, as you do now.

+ Keep the hearth or circle of bricks well tended with flowers, evergreens and fruit, and leave the ritual substances in place, lighting the candle and incense whenever the family or your lover comes home after an absence, replacing them when they burn low. You can repeat the ritual if you or anyone else you love is going away or is facing a difficult situation.

Later Winter Energies

Later winter energies, which run from around December 21, according to the calendar, until January 31, are good for all practical matters in a relationship, home, money, respective careers, for love in the later years, and also for letting go gently if parting is inevitable. These powers can be invoked at any time during the year when questions of security arise.

The Midwinter Solstice or Christmas

The Midwinter Solstice or Shortest Day runs from the Solstice Eve around December 20 for three days. When early tribes saw the Sun at its lowest point and the vegetation dead or dying, they feared that light and life would never return, so they lit bonfires from yule logs, hung torches from trees, and decorated homes with evergreens to persuade the other greenery to grow again. This midwinter magic forms the origins of Christmas festivals throughout the globe. The Mithraic Birth of the Unconquered Sun in Persia was just one pre-Christian festival that was celebrated on December 25. It is therefore a festival for holding on in difficult times, knowing that light will return to your life and relationship, and if there must be an ending to make it as gentle and as positive as possible.

Midwinter Solstice crystals Amazonite, aventurine, blood-stone or malachite.

Flowers, incense and herbs of Midwinter Solstice Bay, cedar, feverfew, holly, juniper, pine and rosemary.

Midwinter Solstice candle colours White, scarlet, brilliant green and gold for cheer on dark days of the soul as well as the year.

Christmas Divination and Love Rituals

These were traditionally carried out either on the Solstice Eve or Christmas Eve.

Sew nine holly leaves to your night clothes and place a gold-coloured ring on your heart or wedding finger before going to bed. You will dream of your future wedding day and see your true love standing beside you.

Tie a sprig of holly to each of the legs of your bed and eat a baked apple before going to sleep. Your true love will speak to you in your dreams.

Three or more unmarried people make a chain of holly, mistletoe and juniper, and between each strand tie an acorn or hazelnut. At midnight they must lock the door and hang the key over the mantelpiece. They should wrap the chain around a log, sprinkle it with oil, salt and earth and burn it on the fire. Each sits around the fire with a prayer book opened at the wedding service. Once the chain is burned, each will see his or her future wife or husband crossing the room.

Dumb cakes, made of oats, barley and water, are baked by young girls on Christmas Eve in silence and placed in the oven late in the evening. At midnight the kitchen door will open and your true love will come and turn the cakes.

A Midwinter Wishing Ritual for Looking to Better Times Ahead

Though this is a midwinter ritual, it can be practised at any time a relationship is under strain due to practical concerns, redundancy, mounting debts, problems with housing, or a feeling of despondency when material concerns and overwork seem to be driving a wedge between partners. Casting money into a wishing well can be used to represent any increase in fortune and appears in countless rituals in different ways as it is one of the archetypal forms of offerings to the Goddess (see 'The Fertility of the Earth' for another wishing ritual).

✦ Begin at dawn on the morning of the Midwinter Solstice or on any other day that is emotionally dark for you and your partner. Take a clear glass bowl and fill it with water. Make a twined wreath of holly and ivy to represent the union of the Holly King and the Ivy Queen and bind it round the water.

✦ Light your first Solstice candle at dawn to persuade light to return to your life as well as to nature, and drop in the water a rich green crystal or glass nugget, making a silent wish for better fortunes.

✦ Leave your candle to burn for a while and then extinguish it, sending the light to the real or symbolic Sun.

✦ At noon, light an even larger Solstice candle and also relight the first, this time dropping a copper coin in the water and making another silent wish. Leave the candles burning for a while and then, as you extinguish them, send the double light to strengthen the Sun.

◆ At dusk, the actual as well as symbolic darkest hour, light an even bigger candle along with the previous two, and this time cast in a silver coin as an offering for your wish.

◆ Leave the candles burning for a little longer before extinguishing them and sending light to the Sun that is no longer visible, an act of faith that better times are ahead.

◆ The following dawn, light the final candle, the largest of all, plus the other three. The darkest hour is past, the light has returned and the Sun is reborn. Cast a gold-coloured coin and make your fourth wish. Leave the candles to burn through, knowing you have turned the corner.

◆ If you perform this ritual with a lover, he or she can cast a crystal and coin into the well at each candle lighting.

TEN

Twin Souls

Our two souls, therefore, which are one
Though I must go, endure not yet
A breach, but an expansion,
Like gold to airy thinness beat.

If they be two, they are two so
As stiff twin compasses are two,
Thy soul the fixed foot, makes no show
To move, but does, if the other do.

[...]

Such wilt thou be to me, who must
Like the other foot, obliquely run;
Thy firmness makes my circle just,
And makes me end, where I begun.

'A Valediction: Forbidding Mourning' by
JOHN DONNE

In Donne's view we are linked to our significant other in death as well as life. In my work as a psychic researcher I have come across several cases where a couple who have been married for many years die within hours or even minutes of each other of totally unrelated illnesses, even when the surviving partner was apparently healthy; in one instance the wife had not known of her husband's death.

Pat from the Isle of Wight told me the following story:

My dad had senile dementia and also suffered with his chest as he'd been a miner. He was admitted to hospital for treatment. My mum was heartbroken. She was in Staffordshire and spent Christmas Day alone. She and my dad were never apart. Not long after, Mum also was taken into hospital with a bad chest. When I visited her she was in a bad way, very breathless and could hardly talk.

I went to see Dad in his hospital and he was getting along well so I didn't tell him how ill Mum was. I needed to get back to the children but I stayed till Mum was on the mend.

I promised, 'I'll come back on Monday,' but Mum insisted, 'No, go back to your family. I'm doing fine.'

And she was better or I would not have left her. The next morning the news came that Dad had suddenly died, and two hours later I heard that Mum was gone as well, though she hadn't been told about Dad.

People may meet and in an instant feel as though they have discovered their missing half, that they have searched all their lives to find; some are even convinced that the relationship existed in a previous incarnation. For example, Jenny had a past life experience in which she was a nurse in London during the Second World War, and recalled how she and her fiancé, a pilot in the RAF, used to walk in Regent's Park in London together. He was killed and Jenny discovered in a later regression that she herself had died when a bomb exploded on her house six weeks after her fiancé's death.

Jenny and David met through a series of coincidences and a chain of unconnected people who seemed to be drawing them together. They experienced instant recognition and six weeks after meeting they moved in together. David had some months earlier experienced a similar regression and had also been previously told by a medium about his life as a pilot. The last time I spoke to Jenny, they were still blissfully happy.

Other twin soul meetings apparently from the past have been more troubled because of present day commitments to other partners, and this is an area fraught with hazards. For while I do not feel that the concept of a twin soul conflicts with the belief I have expressed throughout this book, that we all have a number of potential soul mates, a concept also held by some twin soul protagonists, I know of people who have turned down chances of happiness because a potential partner was not 'the one'.

Relationships based on mutual affection and consideration can be made to work, and passion and love can grow – some husbands and wives have grown together, discovering a deep kinship years into a relationship after what seemed an uninspiring start. Love is not straightforward and exists on many levels, and if you follow the concept of twin souls through, it may be that in this lifetime you need to experience other close kinships, perhaps to learn a lesson. Some of the rituals I suggest in this chapter will, I hope, strengthen and enrich any loving relationship.

Whether or not you accept the concept of reincarnation, the belief that we have a twin soul is one that has existed for thousands of years and still holds credence among those who are either searching for their alter ego, or have found someone who may be of a different generation, perhaps totally unlike them in their philosophy or way of life, with whom nevertheless comes the sense of being complete.

Theories of the Twin Soul

The Greek philosopher Plato described twin souls as follows:

> ... and when one of them meets the other half, the actual half of himself, the pair are lost in an amazement of love and friendship and intimacy and one will not be out of the other's sight even for a moment.

According to Eastern mystical tradition, we were all once part of the joyous unity of the Godhead that contained both male and female. But in order to be aware of both aspects, duality was created, masculine and feminine, light and darkness, and individual but joined souls containing both polarities were created. When we were born, this was divided into two half souls, containing predominantly animus or anima qualities, albeit in varying proportions. These two halves are the twin aspect of the same soul and, so it is said, we have only one twin in the entire universe, whom we may experience as a heterosexual or same-sex union. In the upper realms we also belonged to soul families, and we may meet one of these on earth, even assume different relationships with them in different incarnations to learn different lessons.

So as part of our desire to return to the original spiritual bliss, it is believed that we are all searching for the alter ego who will enable us to feel complete. We may have many soul mates, those with whom we share soul contact, and any one of these will make a good partner. Your own twin soul may never be found, or may take on the role of beloved sister, brother or even a close friend, while others go on to marry or live with their twin soul. For others the separateness that is possible in a less intense love match with a soul mate may be preferable, for a twin soul love match will be very intense and exclusive and this may not be what you want in this lifetime.

There is an ancient legend from the East that I remember reading in a faded illustrated book as a child, that two souls stood on the rim of the world and held hands as they jumped. They floated down to earth on a single parachute made of lotus blossom, still holding hands. But a breeze came and blew them apart so that they landed hundreds of miles away from each other. All they had left was the faded lotus blossom. The man grew up tall and dark and became a prince, while she was born into a poor family and became a weaver of silk, and ultimately wove the dress of his future bride, a grand princess from across the sea, in whose entourage she travelled. In it she wove the lotus blossom which the prince recognised and they were reunited. There was the inevitable pursuit by the angry kings, and the lovers leapt into a fast-flowing river rather than be parted again. They disappeared still holding hands beneath the raging waters, but on the surface floated a single fresh white lotus.

Though it was thirty-five years before I discovered the concept of astrological twins, I still picture them in terms of that legend. Stories of lovers who have to be together no matter what the circumstances abound in literature and mythology, and while some say twin souls are the stuff of fancy, those who have experienced such love confirm that they were drawn together across the miles, and sometimes years.

Twin Souls and Astrology

Astrological twins are defined as two unrelated people born on the same day, at the same hour, in the same world region, who would share almost identical astrological charts. At the strictest definition, true astrological twins are born on the same day within thirty minutes of each other within a radius of 500 miles. But people are also counted as twins if they are born within ninety minutes of each other within a radius of 1,000 miles, or where one or both of the twins has an unknown time of birth but is within the 1,000-mile zone. Because of this there are many recorded instances of astrological twins sharing the same interests, career choices and major life changes. While usually they have similar life partners and tend to correspond to discuss common dilemmas and opportunities, there can occasionally be something deeper when they meet; they may have previously experienced a sense of incomplete destiny and have made love partnerships that failed at similar significant points.

While seeking an astrological twin for the purpose of an emotional relationship is fraught with difficulties, you may find that once you begin to correspond and meet, telepathic links do form; even if you already have or form relationships with other partners, there may always be a close spiritual bond between you and you may become soul mates, best friends and adviser to the other.

If you did become romantically involved with an astrological twin, difficult because you share weaknesses as well as strengths, the relationship would be very special. It may be that romance is most likely to occur for less closely matched astrological twins. You can find astrological twins in astrological magazines, though reputable ones do emphasise that their adverts are for astrological links and are not intended as a dating agency, and via the Internet. In all cases, you need to take the initial precautions that you would do when contacting or meeting anyone unknown for the first time.

A Ritual to Attract Your Twin Soul

This is a more intense version of the traditional candle calling spell suggested on page 33. As with the best rituals, you need very little apart from the natural world and its amazing treasure store of materials and powers. Because you are seeking your twin soul or a soul mate, as opposed to the earlier rituals for someone who would make you happy, a less stringent and some would argue more realistic aim, you may have to be patient if you want to fulfil the ideal criteria for the ritual.

As with all magic, the call to your twin soul comes from your heart, and if, as often happens, the conditions are wrong but your heart tells you it is the right time to carry out the spell, you should improvise with what you have and make your wishes more potent by the intensity of your feelings. There is no Spell-caster General sitting in the cosmos ticking off the listed requirements, so if all you have to hand is a tin bucket and a cold tap, a cloudy night and the nearest tidal water 3,000 miles away, perform your ritual in the confidence that as you do so you are demonstrating the qualities necessary not only to find your twin soul, but to make any relationship work: ingenuity, adaptability, and the refusal to be deterred no matter what the obstacles.

✦ Ideally you will need: a Full Moon; a tide that is about to turn (a tidal river will do, but you can use any flowing water); nine gold coins with holes, for example Spanish twenty-five peseta coins or well-polished Chinese divinatory coins (tiny looped gold earrings are an acceptable substitute); nine white flowers; nine grapes or any other small fruits.

✦ At Full Moon, go to the shore at tide turn during the

evening, ideally when the Moon is shining on the water. Carry your coins, flowers and grapes in a small basket of rushes, raffia or any natural undyed substance. If you have woven the basket yourself so much the better, but if not thread into it nine hairs from your head.

+ Wait until the tide is turning and in a circle of sand with a tiny sandcastle in the centre that will be washed away with the waves, write your name, the date and your wish: *That my twin soul and I may find each other if it is right to be and will cause no hurt to others.* Write the words in a spiral of letters around the base of the castle, using a stick found on the beach.

+ At tide turn, set the basket afloat on the seventh wave, saying:

Twin soul, if it is to be
Find your way back home to me;
Health I send and wealth and flowers,
To the mighty sea, that hours
From now this offering reach
My waiting soul twin on a beach
Far away or nearer lands,
Come O love and take my hands.

+ Wait until the fourteenth wave and hold your hands high above your head and then outstretched towards the sea. You will feel the breeze rippling them and perhaps the gossamer touch of your twin from across the waves.

Where Was It We Last Met?

Twin souls are said to come together in only some lifetimes as they may have lessons to learn alone. Equally, according to some past life theorists, you may be paired in this incarnation with what is called a 'Karmic soul mate', kindred spirits who meet in one or more lifetimes to heal something from a past life or previous lives, or to learn something that can only be experienced through a close relationship. If you accept this theory, it can be one way of explaining and hopefully resolving seemingly inexplicable anger, jealousy or resentment. But even if you feel this is fanciful, carrying out past life work with a lover, especially at a time when you have a problem to resolve, can symbolically explain feelings and help you to work through them, using the imagery of another couple in another age.

Jenny and David's story on page 190 is one that suggests the reunion of previously united twin souls, while the following account from Celia is complicated by present and maybe past conflicts of loyalties.

Celia is in her mid-forties with a husband who has grown distant and a teenage son. On a visit with her local church group to the religious sites of Andalucia she became friendly with Peter, an American living in Spain who had helped to arrange the tour. Separately they experienced past life flashbacks to a period when he was a priest in Granada and she a nun, and they met secretly in the Church of San Christobel. They felt guilty that they were breaking their vows to the Church, but were unable to deny the power of their feelings for each other and planned to run away together across the border to France where there were Protestants who would accept their marriage.

One day, standing near the image of Santa Maria with the light streaming through the windows on to her halo, they both simultaneously experienced the scene in which they were discovered, dragged apart and tortured. Peter and Celia were so shaken, they returned to the hotel and late that night they made love for the first time, though he was almost twenty years younger and about to leave for America to train as a priest.

The relationship continued during the tour. Celia found herself pregnant a month after returning home but she felt unable to inflict unhappiness on her husband and son, although Peter begged her to join him with the baby in America. She decided after much heartache to have an abortion and is continuing her family life, having severed contact with Peter. Many months later I am still working through the experience with Celia.

Cynics would say that the past life experiences provided justification for an affair that Celia would not otherwise have embarked on, but having met Celia she is an intelligent, down-to-earth woman who was totally shaken by the intensity of the past life experiences, the first she had ever encountered. Nor would it seem logical for Peter, about to become a priest, to want an older wife and baby at such a crucial change point, unless he believed it was unresolved business from the past that he needed to finish. Even as metaphors, the past life images expressed many underlying, unresolved issues in both their current lives. Celia does not regret the experience and is using it to rework her future rather than continue in a sterile situation. To follow what seems to be a past life link in this world may not be without cost, so tread softly if your twin soul is already married or has children with another partner.

Within a relationship, past life work can be very fruitful in resolving unexpressed or even unacknowledged feelings. The following ritual works well with existing partners and lovers and can sometimes deepen a relationship that is moving towards commitment.

A Candle Past Life Ritual

+ Light a large beeswax candle after dark and place it in the centre of a table. Sit facing your lover or partner so that the candle is between you and the rest of the room is in darkness.

+ Leave a window open or use an electric fan so that the candle flickers, casting shadows on the walls.

+ Ask your lover: 'Where was it we last met?' and look through the flame and beyond him or her into the shadowy room. Sit silently until one of you sees a scene in the shadows and begins to talk.

+ Fill in the details as you too begin to share the vision, and listen to what the other is perceiving, which may be externally or in the mind's eye, so that like a developing photograph colours become more vivid, objects more solid, and you gradually create a joint scene.

+ Do you smell any special fragrances, hear any sounds – bells, ships' hooters, distant trains or trams?

+ Describe any people you see and between you interpret their words. Continue the dialogue, moving within the created scene if you wish, into other rooms, outdoors or using a boat or horse on which to travel.

+ Do not try to force the descriptions, but build up the puzzle piece by piece and you may find that you are addressing each other in an unfamiliar style, using vocabulary that feels alien to the modern world and yet right for you to speak at this time. The scene will usually not be anything dramatic, for the majority of lives past and present consist of everyday situations and actions.

◆ When the scene begins to fade, look at each other through the flame and you may imperceptibly see another face, yet one that is so familiar that it and your present-day lover merge into one.

◆ Sit quietly in the candlelight and talk over what you have seen, retelling the story of the lovers or the husband and wife whose lives you momentarily shared and who are in some way, symbolically if not actually, a part of what you are and will be.

◆ Some will say you made up the scene and in a sense you did, as it began as all psychic work does in the imagination that is fed by the soul, the past, and by all the myths and legends we acquire from many cultures that are themselves expressions of universal truths. We all share the past through the genes we inherit from our ancestors, and in this rich web of bygone years we can find echoes of present relationships and solutions to present dilemmas. We cannot prove that what we experience in such moments is an actual shared past life, but what we know is that each relationship carries in it many other relationships stretching back thousands of years, and that love is not bound by time and space.

◆ When you are ready, blow out the candle with its gentle honeyed fragrance and send the light to generations yet unborn, whom you carry in your cells and in your soul.

Telepathic Communication Between Partners and Lovers

Telepathy between lovers and husbands and wives is second in incidence only to that between mothers and children.

Telepathy is defined as the transmission of ideas, thoughts, feelings and sensations from one person to another without words, and comes from the Greek *tele* (distant) and *pathe* (occurrence or feeling). Though it is one of the most explored psychic phenomena, it is not amenable to testing, although there have been successes under laboratory conditions, precisely because it is rooted in human emotion, especially love, and tends to operate in the context of the lives of those who communicate without spoken words.

I found Adrian's story in an old pile of research records. He recalled:

> In 1917 I was piloting an Avro aeroplane in the Royal Flying Corps at Dover and I switched off the engine to glide down. The plane entered a strong wind from the sea and was blown into a flat spinning nose-dive and this I knew to be fatal. I switched on the engine and to my horror it failed to start up. I realised that in another moment the plane would crash and I would become pulp and ashes. I thought of my wife Rose and she loomed up before me and instantly the engine started up again.
>
> The very next morning I received a letter from my wife asking if something terrible had happened to me as she was suddenly moved to go down on her knees and pray for me. The time she mentioned coincided with the time she loomed up before me, when I believed I was about to be killed.

This remains the most dramatic example of telepathy between a couple that I have encountered, although I have in the course of my research come across hundreds of cases of telepathy between partners. Not all links between couples are so dramatic. Much of the telepathic communication between partners concerns everyday issues. For example, Mike who lives in Harrow near London told me how one evening he had stopped on the way home from work for a quick drink with Barry, a friend he'd bumped into in London. Mike hadn't seen Barry for years because his wife Julie didn't like Barry as she thought he'd lead Mike off the straight and narrow. When Mike got home Julie was waiting. She ignored his excuses about the delay at work and the missed trains. 'Don't tell me lies. You've been drinking with Barry.'

Mike wasn't surprised by his wife's 'magical' powers. His own parents ran a shop when he was a child and his mother would send telepathic messages to his father if she was at home and needed a loaf of bread or some cheese.

These are spontaneous examples, but it is quite possible to develop what is a perfectly natural channel of communication; in the days before telephones were widespread this was the natural way in which couples kept in touch when apart. This power can still be seen among the few indigenous peoples whose way of life has been unaffected by technology and is manifest not only between partners, but also between mother and children and siblings.

Once the telepathic channel is in operation, you can also use it as a psychic shopping list! Equally, if you are going to be late and cannot get in touch with your partner, communicate telepathically. When you are together, spend time silently talking to each other in your minds and you may find that you can continue the conversation in words, even if it was not a topic you had previously mentioned. If not, all you need is practice.

Strengthening the Link

Telepathy works best through visual channels, so initially visualise the message you wish to send to your partner. Practise one evening a week, preferably on the same day at the same time.

✦ Spend ten minutes in separate rooms on each of the evenings, so that you are not communicating with eye contact or body language.

✦ Remain in separate rooms during the experience to eliminate any sensory cues. Make sure you will be undisturbed and leave the phone on silent answering machine.

✦ Take it in turns to initiate the conversation without words. Choose a topic between you in advance that has many associations, for example holidays or the children, although in time you can allow the subject to be decided spontaneously by the initiator.

✦ Begin by calling the person's name softly in your mind, and as you inwardly verbalise your thoughts visualise a particular scene in your mind's eye in as much detail as possible – the laughter, the rich colours, fragrances, sounds, and above all emotions, for these are the most powerful transmitters of psychic messages.

✦ Write down the message you are sending, along with any impressions you receive in return, so that you do not forget details. If you visualised a place in the message, scribble down a sketch of what you pictured – a cartoon will suffice.

✦ Leave the same gaps in a psychic conversation as you would in an external one.

✦ At the same time, the absent person should be sitting quietly listening and focusing on your message and returning his or her feelings, plus any widening of the topic that naturally occurs. It is important not to try to rationalise the place or name chosen, and if nothing comes, not to force it. This is only a first attempt.

- He or she should write down any words or images received and any general impressions about your contact, especially regarding emotions.

- When you are ready to end the conversation, say goodbye and send a personal message of love.

- Next time reverse roles, so that the other person sends the first message. If you find that you are both simultaneously sending and receiving, this is quite natural, as with any non-psychic conversation, and shows that you are meshing together telepathically.

- Persist for about ten weeks, even if you do not exactly coincide in your messages. After each session compare notes for similarities and there will be more than you expect.

- Of the experiments that are unsuccessful, it may be that your telepathy does not thrive in a test situation. Leave the sessions and instead start to send messages of greeting and love at pre-arranged times during the day when you are apart, and focus on the internal image or a photograph of the other. You can do this during the experimental period if you wish.

- After a while begin to send messages at random times by stopping, sitting quietly and visualising the person in the clothes he or she will be wearing and in their precise setting. Ask your partner to do the same and after a few weeks you will find that you suddenly think of the person you love and the phone will ring.

- Begin to monitor the times and remember to return love when you feel the stirring. Ask your partner if he or she had any strong feelings at a particular time. Retry the experiments if you wish.

◆ Before long you will know if it is a good time to contact a love at work or during an absence, if for example he or she is feeling depressed or anxious. Once the psychic connection is working, a relationship becomes less possessive and tense if a partner is late home. You will know if there is a problem and so free-floating anxiety diminishes as the psychic radar is in place should you need to go to the aid of a partner.

── E L E V E N ──

Sex Magic

S ex magic is sometimes given dark or licentious connotations in popular literature. Yet it is one of the most
beautiful and spiritual, as well as potent, forms of love
magic when practised in total privacy by two people who are
committed to each other, as they re-enact and recreate the
archetypal Sacred Marriage in their rituals.

The Sacred Marriage is one that permeates all cultures,
representing the union of male and female and going back to
the early creation myths. There is the lovely image of Nut,
the Egyptian Sky Goddess, her body made of stars, covering
the prone Geb or Seb the Earth God, who in Heliopolian
creation myths created Osiris, Isis and the darker Egyptian
deities, Seth and Nephthys. But my favourite pairing comes
from the Maori tradition, in which the primal parents, Rangi
the Sky Father and Papa the Earth Mother, were locked in
perpetual embrace. With the birth of their first child,
Tangaroa, it is said that Papa's body became so filled with the
waters of life that they burst forth to make the oceans.
However, Rangi and Papa were so close to each other that
their six children were unable to move or see the light. Tane-
Mahuta, God of the forests, trees, birds and insects, became a
tree, and forced the sky upwards. He clothed his father with
Kohu the God of mist, Ika-Roa, the Milky Way and the

shining stars. Tane-Mahuta then clad his mother with forests, ferns and plants. The sorrow of the parted Rangi and Papa can still be seen in the morning mists ascending from the earth and in the rain descending from the sky.

As the Sky Gods gained supremacy, they married the Earth Goddess who slowly evolved into the patroness of women, marriage and childbirth, for example Odin the Norse All-Father whose wife was Frigg or Frigga, Goddess of women, marriage and motherhood. Her jewelled spinning wheel formed Orion's belt and she was patroness of northern housewives, often being depicted with a distaff. Though such deities were far from faultless even in their own mythologies, they reflected in their continuing union the archetypal unity of mind, body and soul in a permanent love commitment that is reaffirmed not only in annual celebrations of the Sacred Marriage, for example those of Jupiter and Juno in Ancient Rome, but through every act of sacred lovemaking.

The Grail Rite is a version of the Sacred Marriage concept, and one of the most profound ceremonies of commitment. As with all sex magic, if you have joint wishes or needs, you can release these into the cosmos at the point of simultaneous orgasm. Although I write about male and female for simplicity, any of the rituals can easily adapt to a single-sex partnership or the solo practitioner.

☾

THE GRAIL RITUAL

There are many versions of this rite; this particular one centres around the symbolism of the Grail Cup, believed to be that used in the Last Supper, and in which Mary Magdalene caught the blood of Christ. The Grail Cup was variously thought to have been brought to England by Joseph of Arimathea in the first century; transported to France by Mary Magdalene and Sara, her Egyptian maidservant who became Saint Sara of the gypsies; hidden in England in the stronghold of Arthur now thought to be somewhere near Shrewsbury in Shropshire, sent from Rome towards the end of the fifth century to save this and other treasures from the pillaging invaders.

In one of the many versions of the Grail, the Fisher King who was Guardian of the Grail was wounded in the side by a spear, but could not die or his barren land be restored to life except by one who could ask the correct questions about the Grail. The spear symbolises the sacred lance that pierced Jesus's side. In Celtic tradition it is the spear of Lugh, who slew his own grandfather, the old solar God Balor, with it and so brought about the new order.

This is an adaptation of the legend that has fascinated countless generations, in which the question the woman asks is: *Whom does the lance serve?*

The answer is: *You my lady, for evermore, its power and its protection.*

The question concerning the chalice or Grail Cup is: *Whom does the Grail heal?*

The answer is: *You my Lord in joy and in fertility.*

In the subsequent union of lance and chalice, male and female, comes spiritual and physical union and, if you wish, the possibility of conceiving a child if it is right for both of you.

In many cultures, the chalice, which was originally the cauldron, represents the female principle, the nurturing womb, but also the hidden unconscious wisdom, the fierce, wild side of womanhood. The lance or spear, also in some traditions the wand, knife or sword, represents masculine, direct, forceful energies, but also the need to submit to the waters of the chalice to be complete. The chalice represents the Water element in formal magic, just as the spear or wand represents Fire.

For this ritual use a goblet made of glass, crystal, stainless steel or pewter and fill it with red wine or dark grape juice, a symbol of life and in some traditions menstrual blood. Make a small lance or spear from either the oak for power, the blackthorn, tree of courage and of Joseph of Arimathea, or the ash of which Odin's (the Norse father god's) magical spear Gunghir was made, that always aimed true and returned to its owner. Sharpen the end so that it is slightly pointed.

The ritual is very meaningful if carried out by two people before lovemaking, especially if it is the first time they have made love or are marking a deeper commitment in the relationship. But if your partner is worried or uneasy by such a ritual you can perform it alone and recall it in your lovemaking.

Carry out this ritual as close to the Full Moon as you can. I have for ease written the rite from the point of view of the female.

✦ Encircle your bed with branches sprayed silver so that you are enclosed in a tiny forest. If possible, these should come from a fruit or nut tree, symbols of fertility in its widest sense. Leave a small gap in the branches facing the headboard so that you can enter the circle. From the tree hang small apples with stalks tied close to the branches with gold ribbons, and tiny golden baubles and silver bells, gold for the sun and silver for the moon, the alchemical union of King Sol and Queen Luna. Apples are both a Scandinavian and Druidic love and fertility symbol. Around the base of each tree make circles of nuts for marriage and fertility, and facing the bedhead place a semi-circle of pure white candles outside the circle on a table where they will be safe.

✦ You will also need a small round table at the end of the bed covered in a sparkling cloth, for holding items you will use during the ritual. This table should be within the circle of trees.

✦ In front of the candles place the spear to the left and the chalice to the right.

✦ Light alternate candles in total silence, for the only words to be spoken are the Grail questions and responses.

✦ Take the chalice in both hands. Raise the chalice in turn over each of the candles, visualising the candlelight entering the wine. Go into the circle of trees and kneel or sit on the bed holding the chalice.

✦ Your partner now takes the lance in his right hand and holds it point downwards in turn over each candle so that the light may fill it; he enters the circle, placing the lance on the left of the small table within the circle.

✦ He sits or kneels facing you, so that he is to your left.

✦ Hold the chalice upwards to absorb the light from the cosmos and then offer him the chalice. Join hands around it and drink together in silence. Place the chalice to the right within the circle on the small table.

✦ He takes up the lance once more, this time holding it point facing upwards to absorb the light. He returns to the bed with it and offers it to you and you join hands around it. After a few moments, let go and pick up the chalice, facing him once more on the bed as he holds the lance.

✦ He raises the lance above the chalice and you speak for the first time: *Whom does the lance serve?*

✦ He replies: *You my lady, for evermore, its power and its protection.*

- Raise the chalice so that the point of the lance is almost touching it.

- He asks: *Whom does the Grail heal?*

- The answer is: *You my Lord in joy and in fertility.*

- He raises the lance and very lightly touches first your left breast, then the right, the stomach and the womb with the blade.

- Finally, he slowly plunges the lance into the wine nine times and you both ritually chant the Grail questions and answers alternately before each movement; and on the ninth utter as a final chant both questions and responses.

- Place the cup with the lance still inside it on the small table.

- Make love, and at the point of orgasm cry out for a final time the Grail questions and responses.

- Leave the candles to burn through as you lie within your silver wood, pick apples from the trees and nuts from around them, and in true magical tradition absorb the abundance of Mother Earth as a blessing on your relationship.

Sex Magic for Specific Needs and Wishes

As I said at the beginning of the above ritual, at the moment of climax in sacred lovemaking you can call out your desires that will be carried into the cosmos on the release of sexual energies. But you can also focus a sex rite on specific needs. Without being at all moralistic, I do believe from informal counselling work I have done that sex magic is fraught with difficulty unless practised by an established couple. Very experienced witch couples say that their bed is the most powerful temple of all and this is where they carry out their especially focused rituals.

If sex is introduced into ceremonies or rituals, sometimes unwittingly by a group of friends who practise magic skyclad (without clothes), friendships can be strained; actions performed in the urgency and spontaneity of a spell, however noble the focus, can lead to discord and deep embarrassment in the cold light of day.

Sex magic can form a part of lovemaking rather than constitute a separate ritual, even for specific desires. A couple, encircled by candles, chant or silently focus their magical intention with increased intensity and speed while engaging in genital sex, climaxing together and exchanging bodily fluids, consigning their desire to the cosmos with a final cry.

There is no positive wish you cannot make; if you need money to fix the roof or for a special holiday, sex magic can be a potent way of focusing and releasing your innate magical energies so that they can be amplified by joining with the forces of nature and the cosmos. There is nothing wrong in asking for resources to fund joint pleasures such as a holiday or a caravan or car so that it is possible to spend more time together in pleasurable circumstances and thereby enrich a relationship. The old magical laws state that we may ask for 'enough for our needs and a little more'; you are more likely to be granted this rather than a lottery win or luxury for ever, which you might like but do not need. The only proviso is that if the wish is for material acquisition or success for your-selves, the next day you should follow it with a generous gesture or practical kindness to someone else in need.

In some traditions, the couple engage in intercourse, but at the point of ejaculation the man uses the semen to propel the intention of the ritual into the cosmos while the woman brings herself to climax, then joins her partner to end the rite. However, the man/woman mutual exchange of love does seem to me to be most potent of all as the sperm moves towards the ovum, so symbolically spiritually reuniting twin souls as one and spanning dimensions in the magic.

Times and Places for Sex Magic

You can practise sex magic at any time and I have already suggested the Full Moon or indeed any time during the waxing period. The most magical energies occur on one of the traditional love and fertility festivals, for example after sunset on Brigantia Eve, January 31, when you should make love surrounded by a blaze of candles; at midnight on May Eve, April 30, if possible in a forest or wild place, close to but not beneath the fairy hawthorn at the beginning of the Celtic Summer; sunrise on the Longest Day or Midsummer close to an ancient stone circle or standing stone; at one of the later intersections of the year such as Hallowe'en by the fireside of your home; or the more modern New Year, perhaps after love divination or having practised some of the old love spells associated with those magical nights.

If practical, make love in the open air, perhaps in a secluded garden or with the windows open to the sky. Go to high places, to tumuli where earth and sky naturally unite. Also make love in forests, if possible between two oak trees, said to be the entrance to other dimensions, and listen to the oracles spoken in the rustling leaves. If you can find a deserted beach, tide turn is most powerful of all, either at the sea or a tidal river. However far you live from the sea, you can use the nearest sea or tidal river as a marker, making love at high tide, even in a town, accompanied by the music of the ocean will link you with these powerful flows.

Preparing for Sex Magic

+ Try to spend the evening together alone, perhaps walking on darkened hills or through a fragrant garden, and talk of your dreams and joint plans. Be especially gentle and loving. It is important that only positive energies are created, so do not discuss differences or doubts before sex magic.

+ Have a bath in fragrant herbs and oils of love and passion; add a few drops of sandalwood or ylang-ylang to your bath water, or a net with lavender flowers or rose petals hung below the hot tap.

+ Before you make love, sit quietly in star- or candlelight, not touching but breathing as one, and let your bodies join harmoniously with no thought other than love and commitment to each other and to your joint plans.

+ Burn as oil or incense: frankincense for nobility in love; neroli for commitment, for neroli was given to Juno by Jupiter on their marriage; patchouli for sensual love; lavender or rose if there has been a quarrel or sorrow in your lives; cedar or pine to keep out the negativity of others.

+ Light a candle circle at a safe distance from your bed, using gold and silver for solar and lunar energies or green and pink for Venus and love.

+ Softly chant your joint desires and dreams that you would send into the cosmos, and visualise between you the fulfil- ment of these dreams as a three-dimensional image in the air surrounded by swirling rainbow colours that get higher and move into a vortex as the intensity of lovemaking increases.

- Use the moment of climax to call out the wish nine times, and then cry 'It is free' as the energy within your bodies resounds and rebounds to send the symbol now suffused with brilliance and whirling so fast it has become a blur. Picture it breaking free and, like a firework, forming a cascade of golden stars through the night sky, falling to earth as coloured lights.

- Spend time afterwards talking quietly about your future hopes and dreams; do not hurry back to the real world too soon.

- Should your venture be to create a child, you may see gentle lights hovering, even if this is not the night you conceive. As I mentioned before, some parents are convinced that babies are old wise souls who choose them, so open your hearts in love and you may be blessed.

Magic to Increase Passion

If partners have been together many years, the earlier sexual passion will inevitably mellow. But over the years, as external pressures upon the relationship increase and the practical efforts involved in running a home and working eat into the 'couple space' and create exhaustion, sex may be relegated to once a week or month or even cease. When I do phone-ins, older women especially often ask how to restore the magic to an established relationship.

☾

THE BED OF LOVE RITUAL

The following ritual works by creating a magical atmosphere in which passion will be more readily experienced and expressed.

✦ On an evening when you will not be disturbed, light musk incense in the four corners of your bedroom and, an hour before going to bed, take a beeswax candle shaped as an entwined male and female figure. I have seen these on sale quite widely and, unlike red ones, beeswax does not have any voodoo connotations.

✦ On the male figure, gently etch your initials and on the female his initials. Stroke each in turn, from base to centre and then from top to centre for the female and the reverse for the male, using a musk-based anointing oil or, if you prefer, pure olive oil, saying as a mesmeric chant:

Candle glow,
Passion grow,
Wax flow,
Join so
Two are one,
The spell is done.

✦ Light the candle and, leaving it in a safe place, have a bath to which a few drops of ylang-ylang or jasmine oil are added, surrounding your bath tub with tiny pink candles. Swirl the light where it falls on the water, repeating your chant.

✦ Blow out the candle, sending desire to your partner.

✦ Wear something loose and soft rather than overtly erotic so that you feel totally relaxed, and return to the bedroom.

✦ Beginning at the north of the bed, scatter a complete circle of salt round the bed, saying: *I call my love with the power of earth.*

✦ From the east of the bed, circle the bed with the stick of musk incense from the eastern corner of the room, saying: *I call my love with the power of Air.*

◆ From the south of the bed, circle the bed with a pure white candle in a broad-based holder so you do not burn yourself, lit with a taper from the male/female candle, saying: *I call my love with the power of Fire.*

◆ Finally, starting in the west, sprinkle around the bed a complete circle of water in which rose petals have been steeped or to which a couple of drops of rose essential oil or rose essence have been added, saying: *I call my love with the power of Water.*

The ritual works equally well with reluctant female partners. If you cannot obtain a male/female candle, use two separate beeswax ones.

Sacred Sexuality in the Eastern Tradition

The study of sacred sexuality in the Eastern tradition, whether through Hindu Tantric practices or Oriental yang/yin balancing, is complex and I have given suggestions for further reading on page 157. Both traditions regard the human body as a temple, and an act of ritual lovemaking as joining with cosmic and divine processes, a way of transcending time and space and returning to that undifferentiated state of bliss described in 'Twin Souls'. Both use the sexual energies raised during lovemaking, but which are postponed from reaching an initial climax, to unite the male/female energies as the spiritual energy amplified by the sublimated sexual power rises and flows through both bodies as one.

Taoism, which grew from ancient Tantra and has like Confucianism greatly influenced the practice of Oriental Sacred Sex, advocates retaining the male sexual essence, which unlike the female it regards as finite, so that the male ejaculates no more than once a month. However, some more liberated modern Oriental practitioners believe that while you should postpone ejaculation as long as possible during lovemaking, if you wish to exchange bodily as well as spiritual fluids in a final climax, you should do so – this has brought it closer to Tantric practices and made it more acceptable in enhancing equal relationships.

Oriental Sexuality

The integration of spiritual yang and yin, the two halves of Ch'i or the divine life forces that in Taoism permeate all things, in the coming together of male and female sexual energies, creates in the Oriental tradition what is called the Golden Flower. This Golden Flower is a psychological and spiritual centre, somewhat akin to a chakra, in which the subtle seed or etheric semen fertilises the higher or spiritual ovum to create a new essence, of which the actual creation of a child is a manifest form.

In this tradition the energies rise up the *Back* or *Governor* channel from the perineum, up the spine and neck to the base of the skull known as the *jade pillow*, thence to the crown of the head, *Pai H'ui*, and finally down the forehead to end between the bottom of the nose and the upper lip where there is an indentation. The second *Front* or *Functional* channel extends from the tip of the tongue to the throat and down the mid-line of the body to the navel. If you touch the roof of your mouth with your tongue, half an inch behind your front teeth where the palate curves downwards, you will locate the place where back and front channels are said to be united in this system.

Tantric Sexuality

In Tantra, sexual energy is used to ignite the Kundalini, the body's biological life-energy force that resides at the base of the spine or Root chakra, associated with the female polarity of the Shakti or Goddess energy that activates Shiva, the Sky creative force, who enters the body through the Crown chakra in the centre of the head. This Root Shakti earth (or yin in the Chinese system) energy, is raised in lovemaking through 'riding the wave of bliss' to merge with Shiva universal (or the Oriental yang) energy, with the couple experiencing a final cosmic orgasm through the build up of controlled orgasmic contractions; it is said that at this moment their etheric or spirit selves leave the body and merge on the astral plane in a state of evolved spiritual awareness, and ultimately in brief restoration of the undifferentiated state of bliss in which god and goddess, male and female are one. The Tantric system links with the concept of chakras or psychic energy centres throughout the body, of which the Root and Crown chakras form (respectively) the top and bottom of the interconnections.

Sacred Sexuality in a Relationship

Such explanations are a very superficial introduction to concepts that would fill hundreds of pages, and experts in both fields will already have reached a profound understanding of the concept in their sexual as well as spiritual lives. Nevertheless, at any level of understanding, sacred love is a way of expressing the merging of macrocosmic male/female god and goddess energies in the microcosmic human relationship, and however you view the mingling of these spiritual energies as you and a partner are joined physically in love, the result will be the same. The techniques are written in your genes and in your hearts if you allow your natural instincts to lead you.

What is more, absolutely any couple can, by increasing the intensity of sexual bliss slowly and avoiding orgasm until the final release, accumulate energy not only for sex magic, but to share in a cosmic orgasm and thereby experience connection on the spiritual plane.

The first step towards controlling sexual energies so that they will circulate throughout your body before/instead of ejaculation/orgasm is deep breathing.

Prolonging Sexual Ecstasy – Learning to Control Orgasm and Ejaculation

During lovemaking, we are frequently aware that an orgasm is about to begin. One method of control suggested by Tantric practitioners is to allow one or two contractions to build up and then relax by breathing slowly and gazing deeply into your partner's eyes. Relax rather than tense your abdominal muscles and repeat this process many times, so that each time you inch your way towards orgasm you can draw back. In this way the intensity is long, drawn-out and within your control.

Work with your partner to develop this control; experiment changing positions slightly during sexual contact so that neither of you tips over into the involuntary pelvic thrusts that lead to the culmination of the orgasm before you have built up the slow intensity necessary to experience a more intense state of emotional and spiritual as well as physical bliss.

If you have an involuntary orgasm or ejaculation, glory in it; you have not failed because all true lovemaking offers spiritual union and this is a technique that may take months to master and can only be learned by trial and pleasurable error.

One of the oldest Taoist techniques to prevent ejaculation, practised for nearly 3,000 years, that you can combine with Tantric methods, involves a man or his partner pressing a physical trigger point that controls ejaculation immediately before the moment of climax. Just in front of the anus in the male, there is an indentation. Push upwards using the first joint of the finger to make contact with the pubococcygeus or PC muscle, part of a group of pelvic muscles that run from the male pubic bone through to the tail bone or coccyx at the back. The PC muscle surrounds the prostate through which the semen passes before ejaculation. At the same time contract these muscles.

These measures should prevent ejaculation, but not hinder the experience of sexual pleasure.

Gradually, by trial and error, you may prolong the period of gently increasing power and eventually you will manage twenty minutes or more of sexual pleasure before culmination or the ebbing of desire. It is said by some Tantric experts that you need forty minutes before achieving the state of spiritual ecstasy, but others reach this much sooner. Rest if you become tired.

In time you will also learn how to guide and control the other's sexual feelings automatically, and you are then moving closer to total harmony. As a result of increased control, you may experience orgasmic feelings without contractions and may sometimes decide not to proceed to the ejaculation stage. The latter process, a gentle ebbing back to earth, renewed in body and spirit, can be as fulfilling as a technicoloured climax.

Practising Sacred Sex

Do not attempt to make all your lovemaking sacred, but preserve this for special, uninterrupted times or those when you need to feel especially close, perhaps because of external pressures on the relationship. There will be many occasions when you do not want either to postpone orgasm or to impose structure on pure, spontaneous passion. Sacred sexuality is in both Oriental and Tantric disciplines part of a complex path to spirituality, and so unless you want to follow these, adapt the techniques as a way of exploring the deeper levels of love within your relationship.

Try to spend time together alone before sacred lovemaking and avoid discussing any practical problems or contentious issues. If you are at home, put all phones and faxes on hold for several hours. Eat and drink foods of love sparingly: strawberries, oysters, asparagus, quails' eggs, tiny cherry tomatoes. Give each other a massage using lavender essential oil, diluted as five drops of oil in 30ml of a carrier oil such as sweet almond. Warm the oil gently over a container of warm water. Use gentle circular strokes.

✦ When you are both are aroused, lie or stand so that you are not quite touching and look deeply into each other's eyes while you begin slow, gentle breathing, then touch each other lightly, still maintaining intense eye contact.

✦ Exchange energy first through touching tongues, then through heart to breast contact as the energies mount.

✦ Send love to the other person through eye and skin contact.

✦ The penis can now enter the vagina using slow, deep circular movements rather than thrusts to circulate the energies.

✦ When you feel that you are about to tip over into involuntary climax, begin to breathe slowly and deeply and use one of the suggested methods to reduce the intensity. It can help if the man temporarily withdraws his penis so that only the tip is touching the vagina.

✦ At this point the woman concentrates on raising her own incipient orgasm from the vagina and clitoris, so that she draws the pulsating energy via the spine in any way she visualises it as travelling around her body so that the wave of pleasure spreads through the whole body.

✦ At the same time the man squeezes his anal muscles and draws the energy up the spine to the head so that the desire to ejaculate decreases, but his orgasmic energies spread throughout his body. The erection may decrease but this will allow blood to circulate through the system and it will increase again, allowing him to re-enter his partner for the next wave.

✦ Continue the slow inhalation and exhalation of breath so that you can co-ordinate your energy cycles, forming as it were a single bodily circuit, with an interchange of spiritual energies through tongue, breast, heart, genitals (though not through ejaculation), at any connection point, so that the two systems are pulsating as one, breathing as one and merging so that the physical union is only the intermediary of the higher levels of contact now being experienced.

✦ You can either continue and increase the waves of physical sensation until they gradually subside, or decide to end in a physical climax.

✦ At first these deliberately invoked controls may seem to hinder spirituality and spontaneous sexuality, but in time will become automatic. As they do you will find that you may share, not only in the final moments but during the whole experience, what is described as an 'out-of-body' state, where colours are vivid, fragrances rich and you may see yourselves riding across the sea on a rainbow boat, flying through multi-coloured clouds, diving deep among shoals of fish in an azure ocean, or reaching the stars, exploring together flower-filled gardens in lands suffused with light. You may experience not only intense bliss but gradually a merging of specific emotions into a sense of unity, so that you may feel your partner's heartbeat as though it were your own and then cease to be aware of the physical bodies at all.

✦ Afterwards, lie quietly, sharing the precious moments, re-creating your sensations in words.

A Treasury of Love

This Appendix is intended as an instant reference to many of the things you need to know to create your own love and fertility magic. It is divided into sections and can form the basis for your own almanac. Some key substances for love magic are listed in more than one section, but the meaning is always very similar. Each table represents some of the traditional associations and meanings connected with love, including crystals, flowers, incenses, herbs, oils and trees, so that you can create your own love rituals. I have also given traditional candle colour meanings, astrological love links and times that are especially magical for spells and mantras.

Flowers of Love and Fertility

Flower	Magical quality
Acacia	Hidden emotions, secrets.
Acorn	Not strictly a flower, but used in love spells to bring back a faithless or absent lover. Pick an acorn on a small oak branch, wrap it round an ash sprig, put it under your pillow for three nights, saying 'Acorn cup and ashen key, bring my true love back to me'.

Bluebell	Faithfulness.
Crocus	Flower of young lovers, patience in love.
Cuckoo-flower	Fertility, attracting new love.
Cyclamen	Fertility, protection, desire, partings.
Daisy	Idealistic love, devotion. It is said to be a talisman for all who are pure of heart and loyal in love. A daisy root can bring back an absent lover if placed under a pillow at night.
Dandelion	Divination, wishes, transmitters of love. Blow the seeds from a ripened dandelion head in the direction of a lover to carry your thoughts.
Forget-Me-Not	Fidelity to departed or absent lover, memories of love, the past.
Freesia	For increasing trust.
Geranium	Fertility, gentle love, protection.
Heather	(Red or purple) – passion; white – loyalty in love, luck in love.
Hyacinth	Overcoming opposition in love.
Jasmine	Passion, lunar love magic, prophetic dreams.
Lavender	Lavender flowers or lavender water worn by women attracts love and deters potential harshness by partners. If you place a sprig of lavender beneath your pillow and whisper a wish, you may then dream of your wish coming true. If you do, this will follow in reality.
Lilac	Domestic happiness.
Lily	Purity, breaking negative influences in love.
Lily of the Valley	Fear of revealing love, hidden devotion.
Lotus	Mystery, revealing secrets, sacred sexuality.
Magnolia	Fidelity, idealism, strong principles.
Marigold	Attracting love, married love, also jealousy.

Mimosa	Sensual love.
Myrtle	Marriage, fidelity.
Narcissus	Vanity, self-absorption.
Orchid	Spiritual love, grace, unique worth. Burning the powdered root with musk oil is said to increase sexual passion.
Pansy	Affection, loving thoughts.
Pimpernel	Forgiveness.
Poppy	Fertility, forgetfulness in love.
Primrose	New beginnings, reconciliation.
Rose	All kinds of love psychic powers, healing quarrels, love divination. You can plant a rose on a special love anniversary or the birth of a child, red for a boy and white for a girl.
Snapdragon	Keeping secrets, rekindling lost love.
Sunflower	Patience, unrequited love.
Sweet Pea	Friendship, purity, courage.
Violet	White – secret love; purple – pure love and loyalty.

Incenses of Love and Fertility

Incense	Magical quality
Bay, ruled by the Sun	Healing sorrow, protection against negativity.
Cedar, ruled by Mercury	Cleansing redundant influences and negative thoughts.
Cinnamon, ruled by the Sun	Increases passion.
Cloves, ruled by Jupiter	Love, repelling hostility.
Dragon's Blood, ruled by Mars	Male potency, love magic.

Fern, ruled by Mars	Bringing change and fertility.
Frankincense, ruled by the Sun	Courage joy, strength; good for charging and cleansing tools of love magic.
Juniper, ruled by the Sun	Protection, potency, fertility and cleansing old anger.
Lavender, ruled by Mercury	Love and reconciliation.
Myrrh, ruled by the Moon	Healing, peace and inner harmony. Another cleansing magical incense for love spells.
Rosemary, ruled by the Sun	Love and happy memories, love divination.
Sage, ruled by Jupiter	Wisdom in love and love divination.
Sandalwood, ruled by the Sun	Spiritual love and healing. Also kindling physical love and overcoming lack of desire.

Oils of Love and Fertility

Oil	Magical quality
Chamomile	Kindness in love.
Frankincense	Formal love magic, sex magic, solar love magic, male potency.
Geranium	Attraction, happiness in love.
Jasmine	Lunar love magic, passion.
Lavender	Happiness and gentle love, peace/mending of quarrels.
Lemon	Reviving ailing love.
Marjoram	Lasting love, removing negativity.

Neroli	Long-lasting commitments. Given as orange blossom by Jupiter to Juno on their marriage.
Orange	Marriage, fidelity, fertility.
Patchouli	Sensual love, joy.
Peppermint	Passion, protection from critical outside influences and interference.
Pine	Driving away negativity.
Rose	Affection, devotion, pledging love, happiness, removes anxieties about love relationships.
Rosemary	Remembering love, rekindling old love, divination.
Sandalwood	Spiritual love, aphrodisiac.
Ylang-ylang	Overcomes self-doubt, increases self-esteem, opens person to love, sensuality.

Pregnancy
Avoid the following oils for personal use during pregnancy: angelica, basil, cedarwood, clary sage, fennel, juniper, marjoram, myrrh, rosemary, tarragon, thyme, yarrow.

Photo-toxic oils
The following oils can irritate skin if they are exposed to light and about half of the normal amount of other oils should be used – bergamot, ginger, lemon, lime, mandarin and orange. Avoid direct sunlight for six hours after use.

Herbs of Love and Fertility

In the following table I have only listed those properties linked to love and/or fertility, though the herbs may have many other magical uses.

Herb	Magical quality
Agaric	Fertility.
Aloes, Wood	Spiritual love, overcoming obstacles.
Balm, Lemon	Healing quarrels.
Balm of Gilead	Carried as love amulet; good for love divination and protection.
Basil	Fidelity; a herb for attracting and keeping love. Sprinkling powdered basil over a lover will prevent infidelity.
Bracken/broom	Prophetic dreams, female fertility.
Burdock	Protection against negativity, love and sex magic.
Caraway	An aphrodisiac, preserves fidelity. If you are alone, can attract a new lover.
Catnip	Increase of beauty, happiness in home, fertility charm.
Cinnamon	Passion.
Cinquefoil	Prophetic dreams, especially about love.
Clove	A natural aphrodisiac, attracting love and awakening sexual feelings. For those who have suffered loss, cloves offer solace.
Clover	Protection, love, fidelity, banishing negativity.
Columbine	Courage in love, the lion's herb, retrieves lost love.
Coriander	Used in love sachets and the seeds added to mulled wine as an aphrodisiac.
Cumin	Fidelity.
Dill	Passion, protection against love rivals.
Dock	Fertility.
Dodder	Love divination, love knot magic.

Garlic	Passion, protection from spite and jealousy.
Ginger	Passion, male potency, attracts a wealthy lover.
Ginseng	Love wishes, beauty, passion, increases male sexual potency. Often used as a substitute for mandrake root, which is difficult to obtain in sex magic.
Hibiscus	Passion, love, divination.
Horsetail	Repels spite, fertility.
Ivy	Fidelity.
Juniper	Love, increases male potency, prevents rivals stealing lovers.
Knotweed	Binding lovers or friends, keeping promises.
Lavender	Dreams of love, reconciliation, happiness and peace.
Lemongrass	Repels spite, passion.
Licorice	Passion, fidelity.
Maidenhair	Beauty, love.
Mallow	Stand marsh mallows in your window and they will draw your lover.
Marjoram	Consolation in sorrow.
Meadowsweet	Used in love spells, and also strewn about the home to bring joy to family life.
Mimosa	Protection in love, prophetic dreams of love.
Mint	Increasing sexual desire, healing, banishing malevolence.
Moonwort	Love magic associated with phases of the Moon.
Parsley	Encourages fertility, love and passion, a

lover cutting parsley is said to cut through his or her love bond, so pull it up and shred by hand for cooking.

Rose	Romance, enchantment, increases psychic powers, love divination.
Rosemary	Rosemary or elf leaf is a herb of passion, love and healing; poppets or dolls filled with rosemary attract lovers and bring healing. Can be a gentle herb in difficult periods in a relationship, encouraging fidelity and forgiveness, recalling happier times past, and those to come.
Rue	Banishes regrets and redundant guilt or anger.
Sage	Mature love, wisdom in love, love divination.
St Johns Wort	Love and fertility spells, love divination, happiness. Gathered on Midsummer Eve, it is a Summer Solstice herb.
Tansy	Conception and pregnancy.
Thyme	Prophetic dreams, love divination, love in later years, courage.
Vanilla	Lasting love and permanent relationships.
Vervain	A herb of fidelity, can be exchanged with a friend or lover as a promise of truth at all times. Not always easy to fulfil, but ultimately the only way to banish suspicion and the efforts of outsiders to sour love.
Vetivert	Breaks a run of bad luck in love, protects against all negativity and prevents rivals stealing lovers.
Witch Hazel	Mends broken hearts and relationships, heals the pains of unrequited or faithless love and offers protection against all harm.

Yarrow	A herb of enduring love, said to keep a couple together for at least seven years and so given to newly weds and used in love charms. Married couples keep the herb in a special sachet and replace it just before seven years is over, and continue to do so throughout married life – this can be made into a ceremony of renewal. Alternatively, hang a ring of dried yarrow over the marital bed and replace when necessary.
Yellow Evening Primrose	Finding lost love, restoring the balance in a relationship.

Trees of Love and Fertility

Trees have many associated energies, but I have only listed those trees and their properties that specifically apply to love and fertility.

Tree	Magical quality
Almond	Love without limits
Apple	Fertility, love.
Avocado	Desire, increase of beauty.
Banana	Fertility, male potency.
Birch	New beginnings, lunar workings.
Cedar	Faithful lovers.
Cherry	New love.
Coconut	Symbol of fertility and motherhood, the shell representing the womb, and the milk the flow of new life and energies.
Cypress	Long life, healing and comfort in sorrow.
Fig	Tree of creativity, creation and fertility.

Fir	The Christmas tree, and so a tree of birth, the return of light and new beginnings.
Hawthorn	Male potency.
Hazel	Fertility.
Holly	King of the waning year; represents the married male.
Ivy	Queen to the Holly King; represents fidelity, female married love, relationships, constancy.
Mistletoe	Known to the Druids as the all-healer. Peace, love and purity, also fertility and sexual potency.
Olive	Peace and reconciliation, forgiveness, fertility.
Orange	Love, abundance, marriage, fertility.
Palm, Date	Fertility, potency.
Peach	Marriage and birth, abundance, happiness, fertility.
Pear	New life, health, women and fertility.
Tamarind	Love, especially new love and the rebuilding of trust.
Vine	Rebirth and renewal, joy, ecstasy.
Walnut	Fertility, granting of wishes.
Willow	A Moon tree. Intuition, Moon magic, healing, making wishes come true, understanding emotions of others.

Gems and Crystals of Love

I have only referred to the love associations of crystals, but they have many magical and healing properties. Carrying or wearing any of the following crystals will bring you luck in love. Charge your crystal by sprinkling it with water in which you have mixed a few grains of salt, pass it through a cleansing incense such as myrrh and through pure white candle flame. To cleanse the crystal or recharge it, place it under running water and leave it to dry in sunlight, or keep it in spring water for two or three days with a large chunk of unpolished amethyst or rose quartz, making sure they do not touch.

Amber   This petrified tree resin can be up to 50 million years old and may contain the remains of plants, insects and even lizards. Because of its great antiquity and soft, warm touch, it is said to contain the power of many suns and so is able to absorb negativity and protect the user from harm. It will also melt any emotional or physical rigidity within, so it is good for reconciling major differences and quarrels and for twin soul work, especially if you feel that you and a partner have been connected in a past life. It is a sacred stone of love and fertility.

Amethyst   The stone of St Valentine and so of young lovers. Amethyst was a beautiful maiden who attracted the unwelcome attention of Bacchus, the God of wine; Diana saved her by turning her into the gleaming gem and henceforward Baachus accepted the sobering powers of amethyst and it became a stone of moderation against excesses of all kinds.

Aquamarine   This Latin name means 'water of the sea' and it is the stone of Aphrodite and so is excellent for all forms of sea love magic or any in which Aphrodite is invoked. It is a stone for communication, self-awareness, confidence and happiness and so is a good stone to carry or wear, especially for speaking the truth in your heart. It promotes tolerance in difficult situations and, like rose quartz, aquamarine comforts those who are experiencing intense grief, so is good for mending quarrels or facing love sorrows. Also called the stone of happy marriage and a traditional gift from groom to bride on their wedding day.

Diamonds   Diamonds are lucky stones (except for very large ones), symbolising beauty, virtue, innocence and purity. Since Victorian times they have been used in engagement rings. Diamonds encourage fidelity in love and increase sexuality and fertility.

Emerald   Because of its association with Venus, Goddess of love, emeralds were for many centuries worn by women to attract a mate. As a stone of Isis in her role of Mother Goddess, it protects pregnant women if worn over the heart. It opens the Heart chakra to encourage harmony, patience, love, meaningful relationships, fidelity and abundance. As a stone of married love, it also makes a good gift on the birth of a first child.

Garnet A stone of fertility, it stimulates sexuality and passion. A gem of constancy, it is therefore often a token between those who must be apart and is also potent in an engagement ring, especially if the engagement is prolonged.

Jade Jade is the stone of gentle love and because of its link with immortality in the Oriental world, it is associated with past life and twin soul work. Jade offers emotional balance, altruism in love and helps lovers to accept the other's faults. Jade butterflies are given by lovers to their sweethearts at betrothal. Associated with rain, it is also an amulet against male infertility and potency problems.

Moonstone or Selenite Moonstone is believed to absorb the powers of the Moon, becoming deeper in colour, more translucent and more powerful for love magic as the Moon waxes until it reaches Full Moon. As the Moon wanes, so the moonstone becomes paler and less potent.

Moonstone is associated with women, the development of anima qualities in a man and with unconscious powers. It heals hormonal problems in both sexes, as well as menstrual and fertility problems. Since the best marriages are said to begin on the Full Moon, moonstones are a good wedding gift, given ten days or so before the nuptials so that they are at their brightest on the wedding day. It is also a good stone to bring estranged lovers together if turned over three times on the crescent moon for the ancient trinity of Osiris, Isis and Horus, their son.

Mother of Pearl Made of the glossy pearly inside of a pearl oyster shell, mother of pearl is a powerful fertility focus relating to all matters connected with maternity, especially if two halves of an oyster shell, one containing a perfectly round pearl, are placed open on a window ledge either from New to Full Moon or from the beginning of the menstrual cycle to ovulation. The pearl womb is then closed until the end of the cycle; if you make love on the days around the Full Moon your body will, over a period of months, get back in tune with the lunar rhythms that control fertility.

Pearl There are two alternative explanations for the origins of pearls. Chinese myth says that the Full Moon once produced so much heavenly dew, the discarded dreams and memories of men on earth, that it fell into the sea. The oysters came to the surface and opened their shells. The dewdrops fell inside and hardened into pearls. Pearls are therefore, as I suggested with Mother of Pearl, connected with the lunar cycles.

Pearls enable the user to accept love and increase inner beauty and radiance. They are also believed to have been created from the tears of Frigga, the Mother Goddess, who wept for her slain son Baldur, the God of ascending light, thus pearls will alleviate sorrows and loss in love. But because they do absorb thoughts and emotions, pearls are difficult to pass on to others once used. Sacred to Isis, some believe that pearls bring most joy to unmarried women.

Rose Quartz Rose quartz, the stone of Venus in her gentler aspects, is the stone of romance and first love, promoting love, family and affection, bringing forgiveness and the mending of quarrels, emotional harmony, healing emotional wounds, especially sorrows left from childhood that may make it hard to trust in love.

Ruby The gem of love, ruby opens the Heart chakra, strengthening the physical and emotional heart, especially when worn close to the heart. It intensifies all emotions, especially love and passion, jealousy and impatience. It is a fertility stone and a gem to be given between married people as it is one of mature love.

Sapphire Said only to keep its colour when worn by those who are true in love and associated with innocence in love, it is excellent as an engagement stone. It is also a stone of fidelity, whether between friends or lovers, and of chastity and purity of thought. Because it is also linked with Apollo and Solomon, like many blue stones it signifies wisdom and so it is a jewel that will mature with the owner.

Topaz Referred to by Cleopatra as the honey stone, topaz is a gem of sensuality, worn in the Middle Ages on a gold bracelet on the left arm, both to avert the evil eye and as a symbol of love without end; the wearer was pledged in fidelity to the giver.

Turquoise Known as a male stone of power in Central America because it could only be worn by warriors, turquoise is regarded as a Sky stone, a manifestation of the Source of Creation, and is therefore a virility and potency stone. It is also a stone of married love and was believed to change colour if a partner was unfaithful.

Variscite A stone of harmony, it is good for overcoming impotence and problems with the male reproductive system, especially those caused by stress. Believed to protect unborn children.

Love Astrology

Astrological Candle Associations

Each sun birth sign is represented by a candle colour or colours. There is a great deal of disagreement about these associations and so I have given the most common in which there is most agreement. As long as you are consistent you can use these or other colours you find listed in different sources, or choose your special, favourite colour to act as your zodiacal candle. The astrological colour sign can be lit in rituals to represent yourself or a lover born in that period. Inscribe the candle with the appropriate sign for love and fertility magic or add your joint zodiacal signs to any general candle in use, perhaps uniting you both in love. Also use the zodiacal candles to add a particular strength to your spell, for example a Leo candle if you need to be courageous because of opposition to your love. When used in this way, the zodiacal candles are always most potent during their own periods.

♈ **Aries**, the Ram (21 March–20 April): Red. A Cardinal (initiating) Fire sign, for all matters of the self and of identity, for rituals of potency and action.

♉ **Taurus**, the Bull (21 April–21 May): Pink. A Fixed (stable) Earth sign, for rituals concerning material matters and security in love; also for patience and caution if the way ahead seems hazardous.

Gemini, the Heavenly Twins (22 May–21 June): Pale grey or yellow. A Mutable (adaptable) Air sign, for love spells concerning communication, choices, adaptability and twin soul work.

Cancer, the Crab (22 June–22 July): Silver. A Cardinal Water sign, for spells concerning the home and family, such as setting up home or starting a family, and so for fertility and permanent commitment, and gentle love and friendship; also, where children are involved.

Leo, the Lion (23 July–23 August): Gold. A Fixed Fire sign, for rituals of courage and male potency, sensual pleasures and love affairs. Sex magic.

Virgo, the Maiden (24 August–22 September): Green. A Mutable Earth sign for spells to heal rifts, for perfect, ideal love and purity and for bringing order to an unresolved love commitment, especially if one partner is already involved with another party.

Libra, the Scales (23 September–23 October): Blue. A Cardinal Air sign for rituals concerning balancing needs and priorities in relationships, harmony and reconciliation.

Scorpio, the Scorpion (24 October–22 November): Burgundy. A Fixed Water sign for passion and sex, secrets, love divination, and for banishing rivals.

Sagittarius, the Archer (23 November–21 December): Orange. A Mutable Fire sign for optimism, for long-distance relationships, for house moves and for attracting a specific lover. Fertility and potency.

Capricorn, the Goat (22 December–20 January): Brown or black. A Cardinal Earth sign, for fidelity and practical support within love, permanent commitments and conventional relationships, perseverance under difficulties, and overcoming legal obstacles to union.

Aquarius, the Water Carrier (21 January–18 February): Indigo. A Fixed Air sign, for detachment from emotional blackmail, less permanent commitments, flirtations and the marriage of minds.

♓ **Pisces**, the Fish (19 February–20 March): White. A Mutable Water sign, for intuitive and telepathic links and empathy between lovers, conflict of interests within a relationship, love divination, dreams of love.

Astrological Compatibility in Love

Sign	Compatible with	Less harmonious with	Stormy with
Aries, Cardinal Fire	Aries, Taurus, Gemini, Leo, Sagittarius, Aquarius, Pisces	Cancer, Libra the opposing sign, Capricorn	Virgo and Scorpio
Taurus, Fixed Earth	Taurus, Gemini, Cancer, Virgo, Capricorn, Pisces, Aries	Leo, Scorpio the opposing sign, Aquarius	Libra and Sagittarius
Gemini, Mutable Air	Gemini, Cancer, Leo, Libra, Aquarius, Aries, Taurus	Virgo, Sagittarius the opposing sign, Pisces	Scorpio and Capricorn
Cancer, Cardinal Water	Cancer, Leo, Virgo, Scorpio, Pisces, Taurus, Gemini	Libra, Capricorn its opposing sign, Aries	Sagittarius and Aquarius
Leo, Fixed Fire	Leo, Virgo, Libra, Sagittarius, Aries, Gemini, Cancer	Scorpio, Aquarius its opposing sign, Taurus	Capricorn and Pisces
Virgo, Mutable Earth	Virgo, Libra, Scorpio, Capricorn, Taurus, Cancer, Leo	Sagittarius, Pisces its opposing sign, Gemini	Aquarius and Aries
Libra, Cardinal Air	Libra, Scorpio, Sagittarius, Aquarius, Gemini, Leo, Virgo	Capricorn, Aries its opposing sign, Cancer	Pisces and Taurus
Scorpio, Fixed Water	Scorpio, Sagittarius, Capricorn, Pisces, Cancer, Virgo, Libra	Aquarius, Taurus its opposing sign, Leo	Aries and Gemini
Sagittarius, Mutable Fire	Sagittarius, Capricorn, Aquarius, Aries, Leo, Libra, Scorpio	Pisces, Gemini its opposing sign, Virgo	Taurus and Cancer
Capricorn, Cardinal Earth	Capricorn, Aquarius, Pisces, Taurus, Virgo, Scorpio, Sagittarius	Aries, Cancer its opposing sign, Libra	Gemini and Leo

Aquarius, Fixed Air	Aquarius, Pisces, Aries, Gemini, Libra, Sagittarius, Capricorn	Taurus, Leo its opposing sign, Scorpio	Cancer and Virgo
Pisces, Mutable Water	Pisces, Aries, Taurus, Cancer, Scorpio, Capricorn, Aquarius	Gemini, Virgo its opposing sign, Sagittarius	Leo and Libra

Performing Magical Rituals

The Days of the Week and their Planetary Associations

Friday is Venus's day and that of the Mother Goddesses, and so it is frequently used for love and fertility spells. However, each day has its own energies that can add different strengths to your love and fertility spells. Each day of the week is associated with one of the original seven planets visible to the naked eye. Since each planet becomes associated with the qualities of the classical deity whose name it bears, each day focuses on a specific area of need. These planetary associations also apply to the magical hours listed in the following section. You can etch the planetary symbols on candles or draw them on love wish spells.

The Sun

Sunday, the day of the Sun, is concerned with new beginnings in love, a sudden burst of energy to clear a stagnant situation, joy, male potency and any solar spells.

The Moon

Monday, the day of the Moon, is concerned with the need to make a choice, especially where there are no clear pointers ahead, love divination, emotions, sex magic involving the seas, any lunar spell and female fertility, animals and children.

Mars

Tuesday, the day of Mars, is concerned with facing opposition in love, passion and sexuality, sex magic and male potency and virility, and banishing negativity.

Mercury

Wednesday, the day of Mercury, is concerned with communication in love, overcoming love rivals and trickery in love, banishing jealousy and relationships where partners spend time apart.

Jupiter

Thursday, the day of Jupiter, is concerned with marriage and formal commitments in love, family matters that affect love, fidelity, idealistic and courtly love, but also sacred sexuality.

Venus

Friday, the day of Venus, is concerned with attracting love, romance, physical beauty, female sexuality, young love and mending quarrels, twin souls.

Saturn

Saturday, the day of Saturn, is concerned with mature love, the ending of love, banishing old regrets, rekindling former loves and patience in love.

The Planetary Hours

The hour of Venus can, of course, be used for all love magic, as can the hour of the Moon, but the other hours can slant the emphasis of the ritual to an overriding need in the relationship, for example Jupiter should be used if marriage is being sought. Many practitioners only take into account planetary hours for very formal rituals or where the matter is of great importance.

- The magical periods are not exact hours from 6am sunrise to 6pm sunset, but are calculated from the actual varying daily sunrise (which you can find in a diary or newspaper) to the actual sunset.

- The period is divided by twelve to give the daytime hours, and so in summer each will be longer than an hour and in winter each will be shorter. The only exception is at the equinoxes when there is equal day and night.

- The sunset to sunrise divided by twelve will give you the night-time hours – again, these will not be exactly sixty minutes but will vary according to the time of year.

- Each of these periods of day and night is ruled by a different planet according to the day of the week on which it falls.

Sunrise to sunset

Add the hours and minutes from sunrise to sunset and divide the total by twelve to give you the periods for each day. If you wish you can calculate a week or a month ahead using the table below – remember to allow for local and regional variations. The first hour period each day at sunrise is ruled by its day planet. As you will see, the planetary order has a regular pattern.

Hour	Sun	Mon	Tues	Wed	Thur	Fri	Sat
1	Sun	Moon	Mars	Mercury	Jupiter	Venus	Saturn
2	Venus	Saturn	Sun	Moon	Mars	Mercury	Jupiter
3	Mercury	Jupiter	Venus	Saturn	Sun	Moon	Mars
4	Moon	Mars	Mercury	Jupiter	Venus	Saturn	Sun
5	Saturn	Sun	Moon	Mars	Mercury	Jupiter	Venus
6	Jupiter	Venus	Saturn	Sun	Moon	Mars	Mercury
7	Mars	Mercury	Jupiter	Venus	Saturn	Sun	Moon
8	Sun	Moon	Mars	Mercury	Jupiter	Venus	Saturn
9	Venus	Saturn	Sun	Moon	Mars	Mercury	Jupiter
10	Mercury	Jupiter	Venus	Saturn	Sun	Moon	Mars
11	Moon	Mars	Mercury	Jupiter	Venus	Saturn	Sun
12	Saturn	Sun	Moon	Mars	Mercury	Jupiter	Venus

Sunset to sunrise

Add the hours and minutes from sunset to sunrise and divide the total by twelve to give you the periods for each day.

Hour	Sun	Mon	Tues	Wed	Thur	Fri	Sat
1	Jupiter	Venus	Saturn	Sun	Moon	Mars	Mercury
2	Mars	Mercury	Jupiter	Venus	Saturn	Sun	Moon
3	Sun	Moon	Mars	Mercury	Jupiter	Venus	Saturn
4	Venus	Saturn	Sun	Moon	Mars	Mercury	Jupiter
5	Mercury	Jupiter	Venus	Saturn	Sun	Moon	Mars
6	Moon	Mars	Mercury	Jupiter	Venus	Saturn	Sun
7	Saturn	Sun	Moon	Mars	Mercury	Jupiter	Venus
8	Jupiter	Venus	Saturn	Sun	Moon	Mars	Mercury
9	Mars	Mercury	Jupiter	Venus	Saturn	Sun	Moon
10	Sun	Moon	Mars	Mercury	Jupiter	Venus	Saturn
11	Venus	Saturn	Sun	Moon	Mars	Mercury	Jupiter
12	Mercury	Jupiter	Venus	Saturn	Sun	Moon	Mars

Candle Colours for Specific Needs in Love Magic

Although green and pink candles are traditionally associated with love, and red and orange with fertility, other candle colours can add different strengths to your work.

White   White candles can be used for a new beginning in love, to attract new love, for a betrothal or firm commitment or for giving a sudden boost to a spell. They can also offer a protective light for spells. Like silver, white is associated with female energies, lunar rituals and with the Goddess, especially the Moon, and so a candle is particularly potent on Mondays. However, white candles can be lit effectively on any day.

Gold   Gold is associated with male energies, with the supreme God in all forms and is most potent on Sundays. Gold is the colour of the Sun and so can be used in sex magic for male potency or virility, for sacred sexuality, and to bring emotional riches and nobility into a relationship.

Silver   Silver is the colour of the Moon and the Moon Goddesses, both Mother and Virgin, the Egyptian Isis, the Greek Artemis and the Roman Diana, and is potent for all forms of love divination, particularly candle divination, rituals of female fertility, dreams and visions of love, and for all love and fertility magic associated with the various phases of the Moon. The best day for silver candle rituals is Monday.

Red   Red is the colour of sexual passion, virility and male potency; red candles increase the life force and thereby aid conception. They can be used for survival matters, physical health and energy, and also for banishing a destructive relationship. Therefore, this is a very powerful candle colour and should be lit for worthy aims only and in a positive frame of mind. It is best used on a Tuesday.

Orange   Orange is another solar colour, a colour of fertility, both physical and mental, self-esteem and confidence, abundance of all kinds and for keeping or re-establishing one's own identity after a destructive love affair. Above all, orange candle rituals are for joy and are best performed on a Sunday.

Yellow   Yellow is for communication and can be used to prevent or put right misunderstandings or unwise words. It is a male potency colour, but can also be used to keep or drive away jealousy and rivals in love. Yellow candle rituals are most potent on a Wednesday.

Green   Green is the colour of Venus, Goddess of love, and is associated with candle rituals for love and for all matters of emotion, sympathy and empathy. It is also the colour of Mother Earth and the Mother Goddess and so is especially good for rituals involving flowers, trees or herbs, for the growth of love and for luck in love. Green candle rites work best on Fridays.

Blue   Blue is the healing colour and the colour of faithful love, marriage, permanent commitments and idealism in love. It also helps when truth is an issue and for expressing true feelings, declaring love and for calming anger. It is another male potency colour. Blue is used most effectively on Thursdays.

Purple   Purple is the colour of spiritual love and of psychic work. Therefore it can be burned for love divination and for rituals of past life/twin soul work, for sacred sex and sex magic, love secrets, healing sorrow, and banishing what lies in the past but still haunts the present. Purple is also best used on Thursdays.

Pink   Pink is associated with Venus's gentler aspects and so pink candle rituals are excellent for the growth of love and trust, romance, affection and friendship, the healing of wounded emotions and the mending of quarrels; they will help to attract new friends and lovers. Pink candles are used on Fridays to best effect.

Brown   Brown candles need not be dull, and like a ploughed field in the autumn Sun can range from a pale fawn to a rich rust or deep golden brown. Brown comes under the auspices of Saturn, Old Father Time, the God of fate and the passage of time. Brown can be used in rituals for more mature love after divorce or bereavement and for happiness in the home. As another colour of Mother Earth, brown candles can act as grounding, balance and protection, giving love foundations and helping where money or financial security is a vital issue. Above all, brown is a nurturing colour and is the natural focus of maternal matters, instincts and acceptance of the faults and weaknesses of others. Brown candle rituals are best performed on Saturdays.

Grey   Grey candles are used in all spells to create an aura of invisibility before going into a potentially threatening or confrontational situation and for smoothing down potential conflict. Grey is also the colour for reaching compromises and for erasing negative feelings and keeping love a secret. Grey candle rituals can be carried out on any day.

Black   Many people do not like using black candles because of their association with black magic, and you can substitute dark blue, dark purple or brown. However, black candles are potent in love banishing magic, for leaving behind old sorrows and redundant relationships, acknowledging grief and for rituals of partings. In a positive sense black is, like brown, the colour of acceptance, whether of a restriction or of the frailties of self and others, and so is a candle colour of forgiveness and letting go. Black is another earth colour. Black candles are best used on a Saturday.

Wedding customs

- The bride must not look at herself fully dressed in a mirror, but must leave off an item of clothing, for example a glove, so that she is not reflected as a married woman in the glass before she actually is, therefore angering passing jealous spirits.

- Yellow wedding veils were worn in Roman times, and in both East and West the bride was required to keep her face covered until the wedding. The original bridal canopy was used so that malevolent influences could not cast an evil eye upon her before the ceremony.

- In Roman tradition ten witnesses were required – five bride maidens and five 'best men' – dressed identically to the bride and groom so that mischievous spirits, who hovered at a distance at all celebrations, would not know which were the happy pair.

- In Anglo-Saxon times, the bridegroom's men would bring the bride to the church and the bride's woman and bride maidens would accompany the groom.

- If the bride hears birdsong as she wakes, her marriage will be free from quarrels.

- If a spider walks over the wedding gown, the couple will be prosperous.

- The bride bouquet also serves as a symbol of plenty and the ferns and greenery were originally ears of corn for fertility. Orange blossom is a Saracen custom, representing chastity and purity.

- The confetti now thrown over a bride was originally wheat or rice so that when the crop grew tall she would be with child. In some cultures such as Ancient Rome and present-day France, nuts are thrown for the same reason. A bride gathers in her bosom as many nuts as she wants children.

- Originally, a garter was thrown by the bride outside the church. Throwing the bouquet works in the same way, transferring the wedded bliss. For those who miss the flowers, walking upstairs backwards eating a piece of wedding cake and sleeping with the crumbs under the pillow will guarantee dreams of the identity of your bridegroom.

- 'Something old, something new, something borrowed, something blue' is an old wedding tradition. The 'old' was traditionally a garter or handkerchief from a happily married woman, so that her happiness would rub off on the new bride. 'Something new' was the wedding gown itself. The 'borrowed' was a piece of gold to symbolise future prosperity and a symbol of the Sun. 'Blue' was often a blue ribbon to represent the power of the Moon to make dreams come true.

- In many cultures, the centrepiece of the wedding feast or breakfast is the wedding cake. Such cakes date back to Roman times when the couple would eat a cake made of flour, water and salt, to ensure that they should never suffer poverty. Gradually, the cakes became richer, although it was not until the seventeenth century that ornamentation was added. The rich contents indicate the good things of life, as with the Christmas pudding – the fruits, grains and spices of the earth. The bride cuts the cake to ensure her fertility. Everyone must eat a piece to strengthen the fertility magic and pieces are sent to absent friends. An unmarried girl should pass a crumb of her piece of cake through a wedding ring three times before putting it under her pillow. She will then dream of her own husband. A bride should keep a piece to ensure her husband remains faithful and a tier is often kept for the christening of their first child.

- In earlier times, the cake plate was broken over the bride's head at the wedding as a symbol of her husband's authority. The number of large fragments were said to indicate the number of children she would bear.

- Throwing or tying shoes to the wedding car dates back to the transfer of authority from father to groom, and also represents responsibility for keeping the bride shod. The bride was often hit over the head with the shoe.

- Running after the bridal car comes from Anglo-Saxon times when tribesmen absconded with brides to avoid paying a dowry and were pursued by her clansmen. They remained hidden for a month or Moon cycle – the honeymoon so named because mead, an aphrodisiac, was drunk every day to make the bride fertile as bees were associated with the Mother Goddess.

- Engagement and wedding rings have been used for about ten thousand years. Legend says Cain, son of Adam, gave the first wedding ring to his wife. Romans had wedding rings, as did the Ancient Egyptians and Greeks. An engagement ring was to mark a female as spoken for if her lover went off to the wars, denoting her as off limits to the sexual advances of other warriors. It was placed on the finger believed to be joined to the heart by an artery, but originally they were worn on the thumb and sometimes attached to a cord if the husband bought his wife. Diamond engagement rings were only introduced with the Victorians; before then they were often agates.

- Kissing in church – in the olden days a couple would make love soon after the ceremony, either witnessed or accompanied by family and friends, to ensure the bridegroom did the deed and that any heirs were legitimate.

- The best man/father speech of the reception was originally done by the jester, again to divert the attention of the gods from the happy couple.

Wedding Anniversaries

At one time, each anniversary represented a different material, often things that the bridal couple would need or, as with the fruit and flowers of the fourth, that represented the addition of children to the family. Now the custom has been reduced to one or two anniversaries, such as silver and golden weddings.

Yet traditional recognition of anniversaries at regular intervals, by those who attended the original wedding, can provide a focus not only for the couple, but for the loving energies and intent of all present. These anniversary gifts need not be expensive. Even a golden wedding can be marked by golden flowers or gifts wrapped in gold paper. Candles can be lit and the couple and those present burn candle wishes or promises for the future. Anniversaries of togetherness can also be celebrated by couples who have lived together for many years. Key anniversaries include:

First Cotton.
Second Paper.
Third Leather.
Fourth Fruit and flowers.
Fifth Wood
Sixth Iron
Seventh Woollen.
Eighth Bronze.
Ninth Pottery.
Tenth Tin.
Eleventh Steel.
Twelfth Silk.
Thirteenth Lace.

Fourteenth Ivory.
Fifteenth Crystal.
Twentieth China.
Twenty-fifth Silver.
Thirtieth Pearl.
Thirty-fifth Coral.
Fortieth Ruby.
Forty-fifth Sapphire.
Fiftieth Gold.
Fifty-fifth Emerald.
Sixtieth Diamond.
Seventy-fifth Diamond or, more recently, platinum.

Index

Alhama de Almeria 19
Alhama de Granada 124
amulets, love or fertility
    creating 8
    charging 9–10
Aphrodite 30–1
Artemis 31
astrological compatibility
    240–1
astrology 238
    days of the week 241–2
    planetary hours 242–4
Avebury Rings 115

Brigid 18, 120, 123

candles
    astrological associations 238
    calling love 32–3
    colours for specific needs
        244–6
    past life ritual 199–200
    visions 27–9
Cerne Abbas 21
    Giant 17, 21, 111–15
clearing the air 88–90
contagious magic 11
crescent moon magic 26

deities of love, calling on
    29–32
Diana 31, 34
doll magic 11
dreaming of love 62–85
    incubation 63–6
    love journal 69–70
    lucid dreaming 67–9
    symbolism 70–85
Durcal, Andalucia 24

Earth Mother 15, 16, 110,
    120, 160
Egypt, Ancient 17, 18, 64
ending love 143–59
    formal divorce ceremony
        155–9
    handparting 151–3
    healing ritual 154–5
    techno spell 147–51
    washing away sorrow 145–6
enhancing self-love and self-
    esteem 4–6
entwining love 91–3
Eros 30

fertility wells 120–4
festivals 7, 160–88

autumn energies 176–81
Autumn Equinox 179
Beltain 170–1
Brigantia 164
Christmas divination 186
early spring energies 163–7
Lammas/Lughnassadh 173,
    176–9
late spring energies 167–70
late summer energies 173–6
Midwinter Solstice 185–6
Samhain 181–5
Spring Equinox 168–70
St Valentine's Day 164–6
summer energies 170–6
Summer Solstice 174–6
Winter energies 181–8
fidelity 90–4
Flora 44
Floral Dance 44
flowers
    giving in person 61
    flower and candle ritual
        39–41
    language of 54–61
    love and fertility 225–7
    meanings 55–9
    seasonal variations 60–1
    using 60
forgiveness ritual 180–1
Full Moon 8

gems and crystals of love
        234–8
Grail ritual 207–11

Hallowe'en 62, 181–5
handfasting 100–8
    a private ceremony 103–8
Hathor 31–2
herbs
    charms 93–4
    love and fertility 229–33

sachets 53–4
Horn Dance 17
Horned God 17, 160

Isis 18
ivy ritual 91–3

Jung, Carl Gustav 25

knot magic 50

lodestone 94
    ritual 35–9
love divination 126–42
    apple 127–8
    Bible and key 128–9
    candle and mirror 138–40
    creating 6
    flower 133–5
    how it works 127
    mirror marriage 137–8
    scrying 140–2
    seed and plant 132–3
    water 135–6

magical place for two 87–8
magnet magic 33–5
Maia 44
Marlowe, Christopher 43
Mother Earth growth ritual
        41–2

New Moon 8
Notre Dame du Gros Ventre
        19

Oriental sexuality 218

poppets 47–51
pot pourri 51–3
potency ritual 124–5
psychic protection 12–14

rituals
    keep loved ones safe 183–5
    male potency ritual 175–6
    Midwinter wishing ritual
       187–8
    nurturing new love 166
    pledging commitment 169
    return of errant lover
       98–100
    stone circle fertility 117–19
    summer ritual for fertility
       172–3
Rollright Stones 116
roses 45
    six rose pathway 45–7

sacred sexuality 217–24
sea ritual, return of errant
    lover 98–100
sentinels of light 12–14
sex magic 206–24
    bed of love ritual 215–17
    preparing 214–15
    Sacred Marriage 206
    sexual ecstasy, prolonging
       220–1
    for specific needs 211–17
    times and places 213
Sheelagh-na-gig 18
Sidney, Sir Philip 1, 95
Song of Solomon 129
spells, how they work 10–12

St Agnes Eve 20–1, 23
St Andrew's Eve 22
St Catherine 21
St Mark's Eve 21
St Valentine's Day 43
synchronicity 25

tantric sexuality 219
Tauret 18
telepathy 200–5
    strengthening the link
       202–5
trees of love and fertility
    233–4
Triple Goddess 17
true love, finding 131
twin souls 189–205
    astrology 193–4
    ritual to attract 195–6
    theories 192–3

unity charms 94–6

Venus 4, 5, 8, 16, 29, 32, 34, 37
    sachet 54
Virgin Mary 19, 120

wedding customs 247–50
well dressing 122
wishing well fertility ritual
    123–4

OTHER BOOKS BY THE CROSSING PRESS

A Complete Guide to Magic and Ritual:
Using the Energy of Nature to Heal Your Life

By Cassandra Eason

Cassandra Eason, a world-renowned psychic, explains how magic can change your life, from attracting love and improving family relationships to encouraging good health and prosperity. Learn how to tap in to the magic of plants, flowers, and essential oils and harness the energy of the sun, moon, and seasons to reverse bad luck, rekindle hope and passion, and trust instinct and inspiration—the most important magic of all.

$16.95 • Paper • ISBN 1-58091-101-3

Complete Guide to Tarot

By Cassandra Eason

Cassandra Eason makes a popular form of divination accessible and inviting, even for beginners and skeptics. She gradually builds to advanced topics, including cleansing a deck, keeping a tarot journal, analyzing complex spreads, and incorporating tarot into practices like the Kabbalah and numerology.

$18.95 • Paper • ISBN 1-58091-068-8

Essential Wicca

by Paul Tuitéan and Estelle Daniels

Focusing on earth, nature, and fertility, the religion embraces the values of learning, sexual equality, and divination. While most books on Wicca address either the solitary practitioner or those in covens, *Essential Wicca* covers all the bases—from core beliefs and practices, basic and group rituals, to festivals and gatherings, holy days, and rites of passage. A glossary with more than 200 entries and over 50 illustrations extends the meaning of the text.

$20.95 • Paper • ISBN 1-58091-099-8

Inner Radiance, Outer Beauty

By Ambika Wauters

Ambika Wauters encourages women to seek and nurture themselves by dismissing unrealistic images of their bodies. She helps them find their archetype of beauty from within and express their inner awareness by transforming their physical appearance. Includes a 21–day program for regaining health and beauty.

$14.95 • Paper • ISBN 1-58091-080-7

OTHER BOOKS BY THE CROSSING PRESS

Lesbian Love Signs: An Astrological Guide

By Aurora

Aurora presents the characteristics and tendencies of women's sun signs, and the specific chemistry of each sign's relationship to other signs.

$8.95 • Paper • ISBN 0-89594-467-7

A Little Book of Altar Magic

By D. J. Conway

This third addition to the successful "A Little Book" series shows us how we, sometimes unknowingly, create altars in our daily surroundings. D. J. Conway offers information on the power and use of colors, and the historic and symbolic meaning of the elements, animals, and objects to help us create magical altars in our personal surroundings.

$9.95 • Paper • ISBN 1-58091-052-1

A Little Book of Candle Magic

By D. J. Conway

D. J. Conway gives a thorough introduction to tapping the reservoirs of magic in candles. She provides chants, meditations, and affirmations to find a mate, achieve enlightenment, or improve life materially and spiritually, and she encourages readers to create their own.

$9.95 • Paper • ISBN 1-58091-043-2

A Little Book of Love Magic

By Patricia Telesco

A cornucopia of lore, magic, and imaginative ritual designed to bring excitement and romance to your life. Patricia Telesco tells us how to use magic to manifest our hopes and dreams for romantic relationships, friendships, family relations, and passions for our work.

$9.95 • Paper • ISBN 0-89594-887-7

A Little Book of Pendulum Magic

By D. J. Conway

Also known as dowsing, pendulum magic is a technique for seeing into the future, whether for information about romance, luck, past lives, or the psychic causes of disease. Step-by-step instructions are given for making pendulums with everything from gemstones and rings to buttons and fishing weights. The author also explains how questions should be asked as well as how answers should be interpreted.

$9.95 • Paper • 1-58091-093-9

OTHER BOOKS BY THE CROSSING PRESS

The Sevenfold Journey:
Reclaiming Mind, Body & Spirit Through the Chakras
by Anodea Judith & Selene Vega

Combining yoga, movement, psychotherapy, and ritual, the authors weave ancient and modern wisdom into a powerful tapestry of techniques for facilitating personal growth and healing.

$18.95 • Paper • ISBN 0-89594-574-6

Spinning Spells, Weaving Wonders:
Modern Magic for Everyday Life
By Patricia Telesco

This essential book of over 300 spells tells how to work with simple, easy-to-find components and focus creative energy to meet daily challenges with awareness, confidence, and humor.

$14.95 • Paper • ISBN 0-89594-803-6

Transforming Body Image: Learning to Love the Body You Have
By Marcia Hutchinson, Ed.D.

Uses step-by-step exercises for self-acceptance to integrate body, mind, and self-image. We recommend every woman read this book.—Ellen Bass and Laura Davis

$14.95 • Paper • ISBN 0-89594-172-4

A Wisewoman's Guide to Spells, Rituals and Goddess Lore
By Elizabeth Brooke

A remarkable compendium of magical lore, psychic skills, and women's mysteries.

$12.95 • Paper • ISBN 0-89594-779-X

To receive a current catalog from The Crossing Press
please call toll-free, 800-777-1048.
Visit our Web site: www. crossingpress.com

www.crossingpress.com

BROWSE through the Crossing Press Web site for information on upcoming titles, new releases, and backlist books including brief summaries, excerpts, author information, reviews, and more.

SHOP our store for all of our books and, coming soon, unusual, interesting, and hard-to-find sideline items related to Crossing's best-selling books!

READ informative articles by Crossing Press authors on all of our major topics of interest.

SIGN UP for our e-mail newsletter to receive late-breaking developments and special promotions from The Crossing Press.